# CHINESE SELF-MASSAGE THERAPY

*The Easy Way to Health*

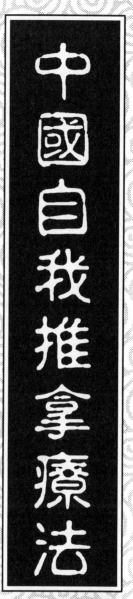

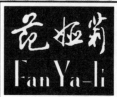

Fan Ya-li

BLUE POPPY PRESS

Published by:

**BLUE POPPY PRESS**
**A Division of Blue Poppy Enterprises, Inc.**
**3450 Penrose Place, Suite 110**
**BOULDER, CO 80301**

**First Edition  January, 1997**
**Second Printing  May, 1999**

ISBN 0-936185-74-0  LC# 96-86693

COMP Designation: Original work using a standard translational terminology

Printed at Johnson Printing, Boulder, CO
Cover design by Bob Schram

10 9 8 7 6 5 4 3 2

# Acknowledgements

First I would like to thank Dr.Vahid Askarpour of St. John's, Newfoundland,Canada who patiently helped me revise my English drafts and supported me in many ways throughout this project.

I would also like to thank Mr. Zhao Yu-rong who drew the illustrations for this work.

F.Y.L.

# Preface

This book is a layperson's guide to Chinese self-massage therapy. Chinese self-massage is at least 2,500 years old. It can be used to promote health and longevity, and it can be used to treat diseases and injuries after they have arisen. Many Western readers may already be familiar with acupressure. This means the application of finger pressure to individual acupuncture points. Chinese self-massage employs acupressure but it also uses many other manipulations, and it treats not only acupuncture points but also other, more generalized areas of the body. Thus acupressure is a part of Chinese self-massage, but Chinese self-massage is more than *and more effective than just acupressure.*

In this book, the reader will find detailed yet simple to apply Chinese self-massage treatments for preventing disease and maintaining health, for beautifying the face and body, and for treating a number of commonly encountered complaints. Chinese self-massage deserves a place in any person's overall health care regime. Chinese self-massage complements and extends the effects of proper diet, adequate exercise *and* adequate rest, and the cultivation of a healthy attitude. In China, self-massage is also often used along with *qi gong* or energy exercises. Chinese self-massage makes a great adjunctive or complementary treatment to acupuncture or Chinese herbal medicine, and it can also be used in combination with modern Western medicine, chiropractic, homeopathic, or naturopathic treatment.

This book is yet another in Blue Poppy Press's series of layperson's primers on Chinese medicine and self-care. In Chinese medicine, prevention has always been recognized as being more effective and important than remedial treatment after a disease is already established. In the *Nei Jing (The Inner Classic)*, the 2,000 year old bible of Chinese medicine, it says that the superior doctor treats disease before it arises, while treating disease after it has occured is likened to digging a well after one has become thirsty. In addition, we at Blue Poppy believe that it is just as important or even more important to teach people how to take care of themselves than to only teach professional practitioners how to care for their patients. Therefore, Fan Ya-li and myself have compiled this book as another way for Western people to reap the benefits of more than 2,500 continuous years of Chinese medical wisdom and experience.

Bob Flaws

# Table of Contents

# Introduction to Chinese Self-massage

## The concept of Chinese self-massage

In China, self-massage is also called health-care massage (*bao jian tui na*), while in ancient times it was known as *dao yin an mo* (abducting and leading massage). Such self-massage therapy has a long history in China, going back literally thousands of years. One can see examples of such *dao yin an mo* exercises and manipulations drawn on the Ma Wang Tui scrolls dating from the Western Han dynasty (206 BC-24 AD). The ancients combined massage manipulations, breathing exercises, and mental relaxation, concentration, and visualization to maximize and restore health to the human body.

In Chinese medicine, health is a function of balance, and self-massage is one simple and free way of maintaining and restoring that balance. It is a basic belief of Chinese medicine that the internal organs of the body are connected to every part of the body by a network of large and small channels. The larger of these channels are called channels and vessels, while the smaller channels are called network vessels. These channels and network vessels are the highways and byways for the circulation and movement of the body's energy, called qi, and blood. This energy or qi and blood is created in the internal organs and then sent out to the rest of the body to nourish and empower it.

Located on these channels and network vessels are certain points, called in the West acupuncture points, where this qi and blood can be easily manipulated by external stimulation. Thus the basis of Chinese self-massage is that by massaging certain areas on the surface of the body, one can stimulate and affect the circulation of qi and blood in the channels and network vessels. Since these channels and network vessels connect with the viscera and bowels on the inside of the body, and since the function of these viscera and bowels is also dependent upon the qi and blood for their function and nourishment, one can affect the function of these viscera and bowels by massaging the outside of the body.

Chinese self-massage is founded on the same theories as traditional Chinese medicine as a whole. These include yin/yang, five phase, viscera and bowel, channel and network vessel, qi and blood, and fluid and humor theories. Although the more one knows about these theories of Chinese medicine, the more one will understand and appreciate the rationale behind the treatments and regimens given in this book, one really does not, however, have to understand all these in order to get the health and healing benefits of Chinese self-massage. Readers who would like to know more about all these theories should see Ted Kaptchuk's *The Web That Has No Weaver: Understanding Chinese Medicine* or Bob Flaws's *Imperial Secrets of Health & Longevity,* or you may listen to Bob Flaws's series of audiotapes, *Chinese Secrets of Health & Longevity* published by Sounds True of Boulder, CO.

## Three reasons to do Chinese self-massage

Depending upon the different purposes of its use, Chinese self-massage can be divided into three types: 1) health preservation self-massage, 2) face and body beautification self-massage, and 3) remedial treatment self-massage.

## 1. Health preservation massage

Chinese self-massage for the purpose of strengthening the body and lengthening life is primarily aimed at middle-aged and older people. The functions of every organ and bowel in the body tend to progressively weaken in middle age and old age, while the tissues constituting the body, such as the bones, muscles, sinews, and joints, also gradually degenerate. The elasticity and flexibility of these body tissues also decline with age. This is similar to an engine whose parts get worn and begin to malfunction after long use. In that case, the engine needs to be repaired in order for it to run smoothly again, and Chinese self-massage is one way of helping the aging body regain its more youthful function and its tissues their elasticity and flexibility. The massage manipulations of Chinese self-massage can improve the functions of all the viscera and bowels of the body and enhance the flexibility and movement of the limbs and joints, thus helping delay the decline of health and prolonging life.

In middle-aged and older people with chronic diseases, Chinese self-massage can both treat disease and retard the aging process. For example, a patient with hypertension or coronary heart disease can dilate their blood vessels, reduce the obstruction of arterial blood flow, and reduce stress on the heart by doing Chinese self-massage. In that case, their heartbeat will become more forceful, their pulse rate will slow, their breathing will deepen, and their blood pressure will drop. Therefore, Chinese self-massage can most definitely play an important role in enhancing immunity and treating disease.

## 2. Face & body beautification self-massage

Everyone wants to be physically attractive and especially people in the prime of their lives. Therefore, Chinese self-massage for the purpose of facial and bodily beautification is mostly aimed at young and middle-aged people. Young and middle-aged people tend to pay much attention to their appearances and seek a strong, handsome bodily form. They also wish to be full of vitality and vigor.

Happily, certain Chinese self-massage manipulations can dilate the subdermal capillaries, accelerate blood circulations, improve the nutrition of the skin, quicken tissue metabolism, and benefit the cutaneous respiratory function. Therefore, Chinese self-massage can change pale and lifeless skin into a healthy, rosy, lustrous glow. Chinese self-massage can also enhance the elasticity of the muscles, make the sweat glands and sebaceous glands secrete unobstructedly, and eliminate aging and dead epithelial cells, thus resulting in smooth, glossy skin, and reduced wrinkles.

Chinese self-massage can effectively reduce fat by accelerating its metabolism at the same time as it regulates the absorption and excretion of the digestive system. On the other hand, for those with weak or sluggish digestions, it can strengthen the digestion, increase gastric secretion, enhance stomach movement, and improve gastric digestive functions and intestinal absorptive functions. This results in improving the appetite and increasing the weight in those who are underweight.

# 3. Remedial massage

When Chinese self-massage is applied to certain acupuncture points, certain acupuncture channels, or certain areas of the body, one can both diagnose one's state of health and give oneself a simple, free, yet effective self-treatment. There are many diseases which cannot be treated effectively by only taking medicine. However, Chinese self-massage is not limited by any conditions. Its only requirement is that one can move their upper limbs relatively normally. After having studied Chinese self-massage and practicing its manipulations, one will see that every part of one's body can be freely massaged by one's own hands, while every acupuncture point on the body can be treated with Chinese self-massage.

In some cases, Chinese self-massage is able to cure certain diseases all by itself, while in other diseases, Chinese self-massage is a very effective, and *free*, adjunctive therapy. With different massage manipulations on certain channels, acupuncture points, and tender points and places, Chinese self-massage can adjust the organic functions of the body and alter pathological states, thus relieving and curing diseases which have already arisen, preventing diseases before they occur, and preserving health.

# The indications & contraindications of Chinese self-massage

Below are just some of the indications of Chinese self-massage.

## 1. Internal medicine diseases

Epigastric pain
Chest pain
Pain under the ribs
Lower abdominal pain
Prolapse of the stomach
Poor appetite
Vomiting
Diarrhea
Constipation
Common cold
Pulmonary emphysema

Cough
Asthma
Headache
Insomnia
Vertigo
Hypertension
Coronary heart disease
Facial paralysis
Gallbladder colic
Diabetes, etc.

## 2. Gynecological diseases

Irregular menstruation
Dysmenorrhea
Amenorrhea
Pelvic inflammation
Profuse leukorrhea

Postpartum separation of the pubic
    symphysis
Mastitis
Fibrocystic breast disease, etc.

## 3. Traumatological & orthopedic diseases

Soft tissue injury
Strain
Dislocation
Subluxation
Cervical, thoracic, and lumbar vertebrae
    diseases
Arthralgia
Sciatica

The sequelae of bone union
Various paralytic conditions, etc.

### 4. Five sense organ diseases

Sore throat                          Styes
Rhinitis                             Nearsightedness, etc.

### 5. Pediatric diseases

Colic                                Poor appetite
Vomiting                             Fever
Diarrhea                             Common cold
Stomachache                          Cough, etc.

# Contraindications

Although Chinese self-massage has wide indications, it cannot treat all diseases. Some of the conditions or diseases for which Chinese self-massage are contraindicated are:

1. Severe organic diseases, extreme weakness, extreme fatigue. When overly hungry or overly satiated, Chinese self-massage should either be applied cautiously or not at all.

2. Certain infectious diseases, such as erysipelas, meningitis, suppurative arthritis, etc.

3. Certain acute infectious diseases, such as hepatitis, tuberculosis, etc.

4. All kinds of hemorrhagic diseases, such as hematochezia, hematuria, hemafecia, etc.

5. On local areas which have been burnt or scalded, etc.

6. Malignant tumors, pyemia, etc.

7. Traumatic bleeding, the early stage of fracture, the initial stage of paraplegia, etc.

8. The lumbosacral area, buttocks, and abdomen are contraindicated for massage during

pregnancy. Massage is inadvisable or should be applied cautiously during the menstrual period. Massage is also contraindicated postpartum or if there is a uterine tumor.

9. Acute rheumatoid spondylitis and arthritis, active rheumatism.

## Key points when doing Chinese self-massage

1. While Chinese self-massaging, the room should be kept at a comfortable temperature, not too hot in summer but warm enough in winter.

2. The fingernails should be trimmed regularly in order to avoid injuring the skin.

3. Except for a few manipulations, such as scrubbing, pushing, and nipping which require direct contact with skin, the manipulations of Chinese self-massage can be performed on the limbs or local areas while covered by soft underclothes or a sheet of soft cotton cloth.

4. During the self-massage session, the person should gently focus their mind on the massage and not be distracted by outside thoughts.

5. It is important to rest after strenuous exercise or excessive fatigue before attempting to do Chinese self-massage.

6. Each Chinese self-massage session should last for 20-40 minutes, once a day or once every other day. When treating remedially, 7-10 treatments equal one course of treatment, and one should rest for 3-5 days between courses.

## Massage media

When doing Chinese self-massage, certain skin-protecting products or medicinal preparations may be applied to the massaged areas in order to lubricate and protect the skin and to improve the curative effect. Such skin-protecting products and medicinal preparations are called massage media. In China, various types of massage media are used:

**1. Ointments:** Ointments are made from medicinals mixed with unguents, such as petroleum jelly or roasted sesame oil. Depending on the nature and functions of the medicinals used in such ointments, different ointments have different curative effects. Commonly used Chinese massage ointments include Tiger Balm and Temple of Heaven Balm.

**2. Scallion & Ginger Juice and Peppermint Juice**: Washed, fresh scallion stalks *and* sliced, fresh ginger are steeped in a suitable amount of 75% alcohol for 24 hours. This is called Scallion & Ginger Juice. Its nature is acrid and warm and it is used remedially for the treatment of cold conditions. It smooths the skin, courses the channels, quickens the blood, dispels cold, and resolves the exterior. It can also be used in winter and spring without there necessarily being symptoms of cold.

Washed peppermint can also be steeped in 75% alcohol. Its nature is acrid and warm. It smooths the skin, clears evil heat, resolves the exterior, removes summerheat, and reduces fever. This is called Peppermint Juice and is used to treat warm or hot conditions. It can also be used in the summer without there necessarily being a hot disease.

**3. Talcum Powder**: Talcum powder can be used all year round. It reduces friction and smooths the skin to prevent chafing.

## Chinese self-massage as an adjunctive therapy

Traditionally in China, self-massage was and is only one part of a holistic lifestyle leading to long life and good health. In order for Chinese self-massage to get its greatest effects, besides perseverance and patience, a healthy diet and proper amounts of rest and exercise are vitally important. For more information on other methods of Chinese medical self-care, the reader should see Bob Flaws's *Arisal of the Clear: A Simple Guide to Healthy Eating According to Traditional Chinese Medicine* and his *Imperial Secrets of Health & Longevity.* As mentioned above, Sounds True Audio has also published a six audiotape series by Bob Flaws titled *Chinese Secrets of Health & Longevity.*

Chinese self-massage may also be used as part of an overall treatment plan for the remedying of particular diseases. Chinese self-massage can be successfully combined with modern Western medicine, chiropractic, homeopathic, and naturopathic medicines. In particular, Chinese self-massage is a wonderful adjunctive therapy for those undergoing a course of acupuncture or Chinese herbal medicine. In that case, one's acupuncturist or Chinese medical practitioner can help select the best and most appropriate manipulations from this book and show the reader where to locate the acupuncture points on their body exactly. When Chinese self-massage is used along with acupuncture and Chinese herbal medicine, it makes those other therapies even more effective and the course of treatment that much shorter.

Chinese medicine is the greatest rising star in the world of alternative or complementary medicine today. This is because people all around the world are realizing that the Chinese have accumulated within their national medicine the combined experience of more than 100 generations of highly trained and literate doctors. Although traditional Chinese medicine contains within it all the wisdom and experience of the Chinese folk, traditional Chinese medicine is not just a folk medicine. In fact, it is the oldest, continually practiced, literate, professional secular medicine in the world today. In comparison, most other medical systems are still in their infancy. For those readers who would like to experience the many healing benefits of professional Chinese medicine, the last chapter in this book gives ideas on how to find a qualified local practitioner.

CHAPTER
2

# Chinese Self-massage for Health Preservation

## Local self-massage

Local self-massage in order to promote the flow of qi, blood, and bodily fluids and therefore improve the nourishment and function of local areas can be carried out on every part of the body. By improving the nourishment and function of the local area, the health of that area is preserved and maximized at the same time as it relieves fatigue and prevents disease.

Local self-massage for health preservation is the oldest of all methods of Chinese self-massage. In antiquity, it was also called "local massage and *gong*-inducing method." *Gong* means a special training exercise or *qi gong*. Most Chinese self-massage methods of ancient times were a combination of breathing exercises and massage movements. In other words, self-massage manipulations were combined with breath regulation and mind concentration in order to regulate the bodily functions. This is based on the realization that the mind moves with the breath and that the body and mind are really the bodymind — a single, integrated entity and not two separate and independent things. Therefore, because of its ancient history, the benefits of Chinese self-massage for health promotion and preservation are well tested and authenticated by countless ancient Chinese doctors over lifetimes of long practice.

As stated above, this type of Chinese self-massage is especially suitable for middle-aged and older persons. However, it can also be used by anyone, including athletes, for relieving fatigue and strain of various body parts due to overuse.

# 1. Self-massage of the head, face, eyes, nose & ears

## A. Self-massage of the head & face

**Massage methods:**

1. Pushing apart the forehead: Place the middle segments of both bent index fingers at the midpoint of the forehead between the two eyes. Then push apart along the eyebrows till the index fingers reach the anterior hairline on the temples.
Repeat this process, moving the index fingers up the forehead progressively with each pushing out movement until one reaches the anterior hairline on the top of the forehead. Then go back down to the level of the eyebrows and again push apart at the level of the eyebrows. Do this 30-50 times altogether.

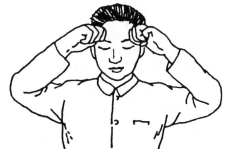

2. Wiping the temples: Press the temples with the pads of the thumbs and wipe backwards repeatedly with force approximately 30 times. For best results, one should create a sensation of mild soreness and distention in the local area.
This mild sensation of soreness and distention shows that the qi or energy has been stimulated and is now filling the local area with nourishing and empowering qi and blood.

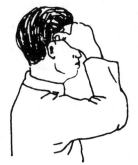

12

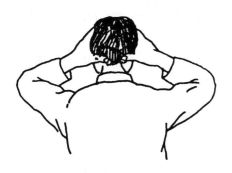

3. Press & knead the back of the head: Place the pads or the tips of both thumbs securely on the points *Feng Chi* (GB 20). This point is located 1 body inch (*i.e.*, approximately the width of the thumb knuckle) above the posterior hairline in the depression between the mastoid process and the long muscles at the back of the neck. Press these forcefully more then 10 times followed by circular kneading. Then knead *Nao Kong* (GB 19, located 1.5 body inches above *Feng Chi*) approximately 30 times. For best effect, one should create a sensation of mild soreness and distention in the local area.

4. Patting the vertex: Sit upright with eyes looking straight ahead and teeth clenched. Then pat the very top of the head rhythmically with the palm approximately 10 times.

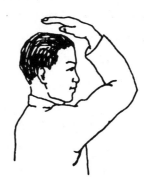

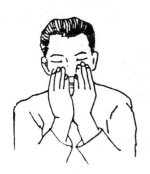

5. Washing the face with the hands: Rub the palms of the hands briskly against each other until they are warm. Then place the palms tightly against the forehead, rubbing forcefully down to the lower jaws and along the edges of the lower jaws beside the points *Jia Che* (St 6, located 1 finger-width anterior and superior to the angle of the jaw). Then continue rubbing on upwards past the fronts of the ears and the temples to the midpoint of the forehead. Repeat this procedure 20-30 times until a warm sensation is felt all over the face.

**Functions & indications:** The above Chinese self-massage techniques invigorate the brain, improve the intelligence, quiet the mind, and calm over-excitement. They can be used for preventing and treating headache, dizziness, insomnia, forgetfulness, neurosis, and facial paralysis. These maneuvers can be done twice a day, once in the morning and once in the afternoon.

## B. Self-massage of the eyes

**Massage methods:**

1. Kneading *Zan Zhu* (Bl 2): Press with the pads of both thumbs on the points *Zan Zhu* (each of which are located in the depressions just medial to the medial ends of the eyebrows), kneading with gradually increasing force approximately 100 times until there is a feeling of mild soreness and distention.

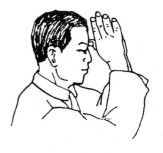

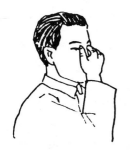

2. Pressing *Jing Ming* (Bl 1): Press with the pads of the thumb and index finger of the right hand on the points *Jing Ming* (each of which is located in the depressions 0.1 body inches anterior and superior to the inner canthi of both eyes). Press down and pinch up alternatively approximately 100 times until there is a feeling of mild soreness and distention.

3. Pressing & kneading *Si Bai* (St 2): Press and knead with the index fingers of both hands on the points *Si Bai* (each of which is located at 1 body inch under the midpoint of the lower orbit of each eye) approximately 100 times until there is a sensation of mild soreness and distention.

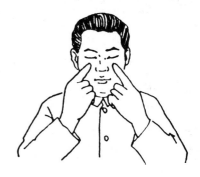

4. Wiping the orbits: Bend the index fingers and wipe with the lateral sides of their middle segments on the upper and then lower orbits from the inner corners of the eyes to the outer 20-30 times.

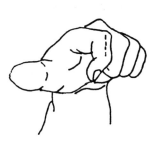
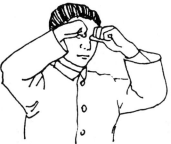
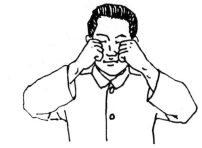

5. Heating the eyes: Close the eyes lightly. Then rub the palms of the hands briskly against each other until they are hot. Then cover the eyes with the palms for about 30-60 seconds, followed by lightly kneading them approximately 10 times.

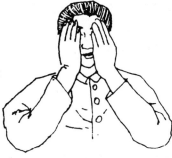

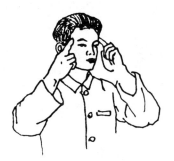

6. Kneading *Tai Yang* (M-HN-9): Press with the tips of the thumbs or middle fingers on the points *Tai Yang* (each of which is located 1 body inch lateral to the lateral end of the eyebrow and the outer canthus) and knead them approximately 100 times until there is a sensation of mild soreness and distention.

**Functions & indications:** These manipulations can be used for preventing and treating myopia, blurred vision, glaucoma, optic nerve atrophy, and other eye diseases. They may also be used to relax the eyes after long hours of reading or for diminished visual acuity in the elderly.

15

## C. Self-massage of the nose

**Massage methods:**

1. Pressing & kneading *Ying Xiang* (LI 20): Press with the pads of the index and middle fingers of one hand on the points *Ying Xiang* (each of which is located 0.5 body inches lateral to the wing of the nose on each side). Press and knead these 50-100 times until there is a mild sensation of soreness and distention.

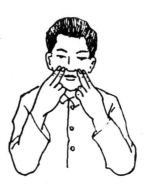

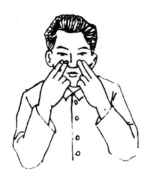

2. Pressing & kneading *Bi Tong* (M-HN-14): Press and knead with the pads of the index and middle fingers of one hand on the points *Bi Tong* (which are lateral to the root of the nose on both sides) 50-100 times until there is a mild sensation of soreness and distention.

3. Rubbing the sides of the nose: Rub the index or middle fingers of both hands against each other until they are hot and then rub them on both sides of the nose approximately 30-50 times up and down until the nose becomes hot as well.

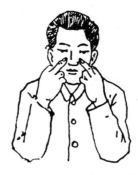

**Functions & indications:** These manipulations can be used for preventing and treating the common cold, stuffy and runny nose, allergic rhinitis, chronic rhinitis, paranasal sinusitis, etc.

## D. Self-massage of the ears

**Massage methods:**

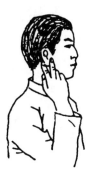

1. Pressing & kneading the points around the ears: Press and knead with the tips of the middle fingers on the points *Er Men* (TB 21, located in front and above the center of the tragus or fleshy tab at the front of the ear), *Ting Gong* (SI 19, located in the middle in front of the tragus), and *Ting Hui* (GB 2, located in front of and below the center of the tragus), and the points *Yi Feng* (TB 17, located in the depression behind the earlobes), 30-50 times each point until there is a mild sensation of soreness and distention.

2. Rubbing the helices: Pinch the helices of both ears gently with the thumbs and the lateral sides of the index fingers, rubbing up and down repeatedly 30-50 times until the helices become hot.

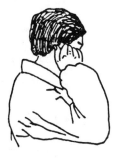

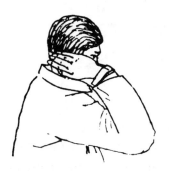

3. Sounding the heavenly drum: Cover both ears with both palms, the bases of the palms pointing to the front and the fingers to the back. Then flick on the protruding bones behind the ears with the index and middle fingers. This flicking is done by placing the middle finger over the index finger and then sliding it quickly down off the index finger. Do this 20-30 times. A booming sound should be produced in the ears.

4. Pressurizing & depressurizing the air inside the ears: Press both ear openings tightly with both palms, making the inner ears full of air. Then loosen them quickly and repeatedly approximately 10 times. The force of pressing and releasing should not be too strong.

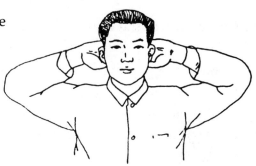

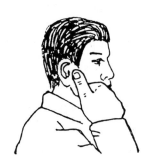

5. Rubbing the area in front of the ears: Place the lateral sides of the two thumbs or the palmar surfaces of the index fingers tightly on the areas in front of the ears, rubbing up and down repeatedly approximately 30 times until a sensation of heat is felt.

**Functions & indications:** These maneuvers can be used for preventing and treating tinnitus, deafness, and otitis media as well as for the care of the health of the ears and the prevention of ear diseases in the elderly.

## 2. Self-massage of the chest & abdomen

### A. Self-massage of the chest

**Massage methods:**

1. Pressing & kneading the chest: Press and knead with the pad of the middle finger on the points *Shan Zhong* (CV 17, located at the midpoint between the nipples), *Zhong Fu* (Lu 1, located 6 body inches lateral to the midline of the chest in the first intercostal space), *Ru Gen* (St 18, located 0.2 body inches inferior to the nipple),

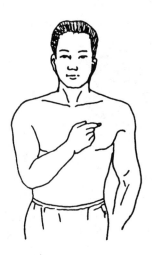

18

and *Ru Pang* (located 0.2 body inches lateral to the nipple). Press and knead each point 30-50 times. Then, starting from the region below the collar - bone, press and knead with fairly hard force every intercostal space from its midline to the sides and from top to bottom till there is a mild sensation of soreness and distention.

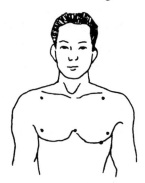

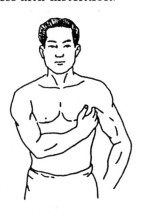

2. Grasping muscles of the thorax: Place one thumb tightly against the opposite side of the chest and the index and middle fingers of the same hand against the side of the chest below the armpit. Lift and grasp the pectoral muscle with force. Breathe in while lifting up and breathe out while relaxing down. Relaxing down should be slow and accompanied by gentle kneading. Repeat this procedure approximately 5 times on each side of the chest. (Fig. 61)

3. Patting the chest: Pat the chest with a hollow palm from top to bottom along the midline of the chest, the median line of the breast, and the median lines under the armpits approximately 10 times each. Be sure not to hold one's breath while doing this patting.

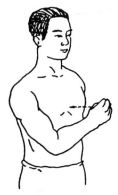

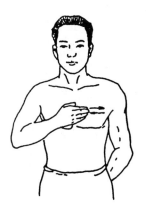

4. Rubbing the chest: Place the large, fleshy pad of muscle at the base of the thumb or the whole palm of one hand tightly against the surface of the chest, rubbing forcefully to and fro transversely approximately 20 times until a warm feeling is produced. However one should avoid rubbing so hard as to cause a skin abrasion.

**Functions & indications:** These manipulations can be used for treating and preventing pain in the chest when breathing, chest pain, a tight feeling in the chest, cough, asthma, etc. The right side of the chest should be massaged with the left hand and the left side with the right hand.

## B. Self-massage of the abdomen

**Massage methods:**

1. Kneading *Zhong Wan* (CV 12): Place the fleshy pad of muscle at the base of the thumb of one hand tightly against the point *Zhong Wan* (midpoint between the navel and the base of the sternum on the midline of the upper abdomen). Then knead clockwise with gentle force for 2-5 minutes.

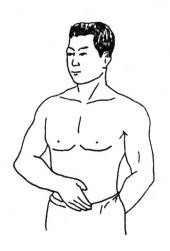

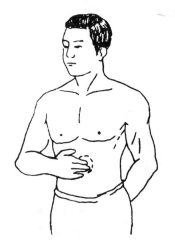

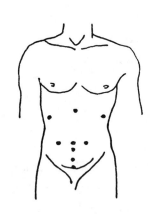

2. Pressing & kneading the points on the abdomen: Press and knead with the tip of the middle finger, the fleshy pad of muscle at the base of the thumb, or the heel of the palm of the hand on the points *Tian Shu* (St 25, 2 body inches lateral to the navel), *Qi Hai* (CV 6, 1.5 body inches inferior to the navel), *Guan Yuan* (CV 4, 3 body inches inferior to the navel), and *Zhong Ji* (CV 3, 4 body inches inferior to the navel) 30-50 times each.

20

3. Circular rubbing the abdomen: Place the hollow of one palm on the navel and with the other palm press on top of the first palm, rubbing circularly with gentle force clockwise for approximately 2-5 minutes.

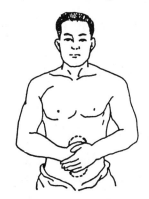

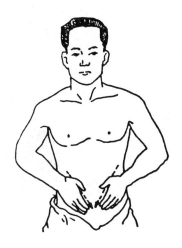

4. Rubbing the lower abdomen: Place the fleshy pad of muscle at the base of the pinkies or little fingers of both hands against the points *Tian Shu* (St 25, 2 body inches lateral to the navel), rubbing up and down approximately 30 times until a warm sensation is felt.

5. Rubbing the lateral costal regions: Place the fleshy pad of muscle at the base of the thumbs of both hands against the area on top of the ribs under the armpits. Rub with force to and fro quickly approximately 30 times or until a warm sensation is felt.

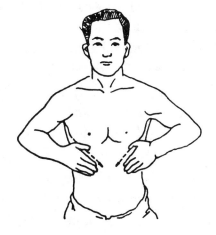

**Functions & indications:** These manipulations can be used for treating and preventing discomfort in the stomach, indigestion, constipation, abdominal pain, diarrhea, irregular menstruation, and impotence.

# 3. Self-massage of the neck, upper back & lumbosacral region

## A. Self-massage of the neck & upper back

**Massage methods:**

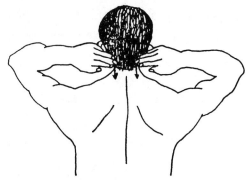

1. Pressing & kneading the neck and upper back: First, use the tips of the index, middle, and ring fingers of both hands to press and knead both sides of the neck and the middle of the nape of the neck from top to bottom 5-10 times for each line. Then press and knead with the middle fingers on the points *Feng Chi* (GB 20, located 1 body inch above the posterior hairline in the depression between the mastoid process and the long muscles at the back of the neck), *Feng Fu* (GV 16, located 1 cun above the middle of the posterior hairline), *Da Zhui* (GV 14, located at the center under the bulging bone at the base of the skull), *Shen Zhu* (GV 12, located at the lower border of the spinous process of the 3rd thoracic vertebra), *Da Zhu* (Bl 11, located 1.5 body inches lateral to the lower border of the spinous process of the 1st thoracic vertebra), *Feng Men* (Bl 12, located 1.5 body inches lateral to the lower border of the spinous process of the 2nd thoracic vertebra),and *Fei Shu* (Bl 13, located 1.5 body inches lateral to the lower border of the spinous process of the 3rd thoracic vertebra) approximately 30 times each.

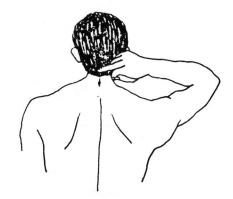

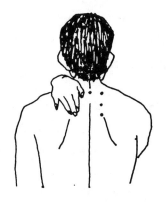

2. Grasping the muscles on both sides of the nape of the neck: Place the thumb of one hand on one side of the back of the neck and the index and middle fingers on the other side, grasping the muscles of both sides from top to bottom 5-10 times.

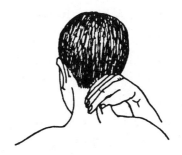

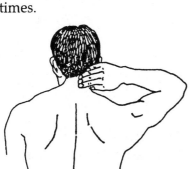

3. Rubbing the neck: Rub with one palm on the middle and both sides of the nape of the neck to and fro 10-20 times for each line until the region becomes hot.

4. Patting the back: With each hollow palm, pat the other side of the back alternately approximately 10 times on each side.

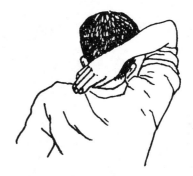

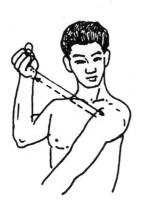

5. Pounding *Jian Jing* (GB 21): Keeping the upper body erect, make an empty fist and pound it on the point *Jian Jing* (midpoint on the top of the shoulder) on the opposite side 20-30 times. Then pound the other *Jian Jing* on the other side of the shoulder with the other fist the same number of times.

6. Circular rubbing *Gao Huang*: Keeping
the upper body erect, bring both arms
up to the sides to form a 90 degree angle.
Bend the elbows. Then rotate the
shoulder joints to the farthest extent
of their backward stretch to stimulate
points such as *Gao Huang Shu* (Bl 43,
located in the interscapular region)
by the rotating movement of the
scapula.

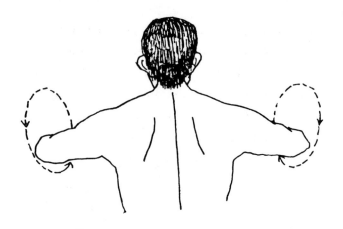

**Functions & indications:** These manipulations can be used for treating and preventing
cervical spondylopathy, stiff neck, pain, soreness, and distention in the upper back, cough,
asthma, stiffness and pain in the chest, heart palpitations, and angina pectoris.

## B. Self-massage of the lumbar region

**Massage methods:**

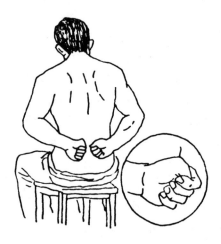

1. Kneading the points at the waist: Clench the fists
and knead with the knuckles of the index fingers on
the paired points *Shen Shu* (Bl 23, located 1.5 body
inches lateral to the lower border of the 2nd lumbar
spinous process), *Zhi Shi* (Bl 52, located 3 body inches
lateral to the lower border of the 2nd lumbar spinous
process), and *Yao Yan* (M-BW-24, located 3- 4 body
inches lateral to the lower border of the 4th lumbar
spinous process) 30-50 times each until there is a mild
sensation of soreness and distention.

2. Pounding the lumbar region: Clench the fists and pound with their tops from top to bottom along the lumbosacral midline, the two lines which are 1.5 body inches lateral to the midline, and the two lines which are 3 body inches lateral to the midline 5-10 times each.

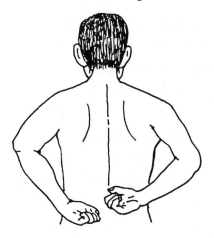

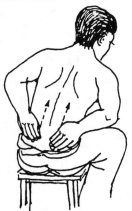

3. Rubbing the waist: Place the two palms tightly on the sides of the waist. Rub the waist up and down forcefully until the region is hot.

4. Moving the waist: Move the waist actively forward, backward, and in a circular rotation.

**Functions & indications:** These manipulations can be used for preventing and treating soreness and pain in the waist, listlessness, insomnia, impotence, irregular menstruation, diarrhea, frequent urination, hyperplasia of the lumbar vertebrae, prolapse of the lumbar intervertebral discs, lumbar muscle strain, etc. They relax the lumbar muscles, relieve fatigue, and strengthen the movement of the waist.

# 4. Self-massage of the extremities

## A. Self-massage of the upper limbs

**Massage methods:**

1. Pressing & kneading the points of the upper limbs: Press and knead with the tip of the thumb or middle finger on the following points in the following order: *(1) Jian Nei Shu* (M-UE-48, located at the front of the shoulder), (2) *Jian Yu* (LI 15, located in the depression lateral to the highest point of the shoulder), and (3) *Jian Jing* (GB 21, located at the midpoint on the top of the shoulder). Rotate the shoulder at same time. Then press and knead the points (4) *Qu Chi* (LI 11, located at the lateral end of the transverse crease when the elbow is flexed), (6) *Shou San Li* (LI 10, located 2 body inches below *Qu Chi*), *Chi Ze* (Lu 5, located in the elbow crease on the radial side of the tendon), *Qu Ze* (Per 3, located in the elbow crease on ulnar side of the tendon), *Shao Hai* (Ht 3, located at the lateral end of the elbow crease when the elbow is flexed), and (5) *Xiao Hai* (SI 8, located in the depression on the inner side of the tip of the elbow when the elbow is flexed). Press and knead the points *Wai Guan* (TB 5, located between the two bones 2 body inches above the wrist crease on the back of the forearm), (7) *Nei Guan* (Per 6, located between the tendons 2 body inches above the wrist crease on the front of the forearm),

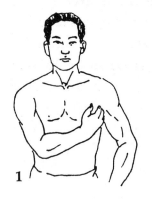
1

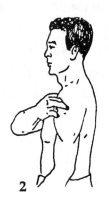
2

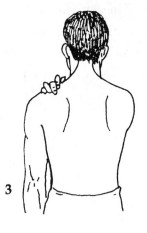
3

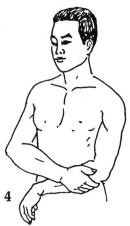
4

*Yang Chi* (TB 4, located on the ulnar side of the tendon in the middle of the crease on the back of the wrist), *Yang Xi* (LI 5, located between the two tendons on the radial side of the crease on the back of the wrist), and (8) *He Gu* (LI 4, located in the fleshy mound in the center of the angle on the back of the hand between the thumb and index fingers). Press and knead each of these points 30- 50 times to produce a feeling of mild soreness and distention.

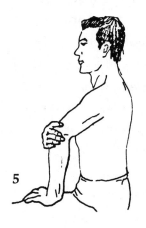

5

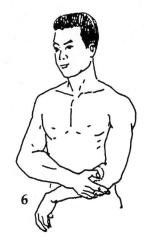

6

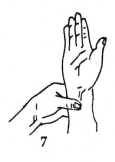

7

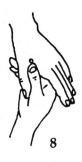

8

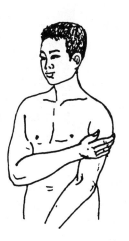

2. Grasping the upper limbs: Using the thumb and the other four fingers of one hand, hold the upper limb on the opposite side. Grasp along the lateral side from the shoulder to the wrist 3-5 times. Then grasp along the medial side from the armpit to the wrist 3-5 times. Grasping, releasing, and moving along the upper limb like this can soothe the muscles and make the upper limb comfortable and relaxed.

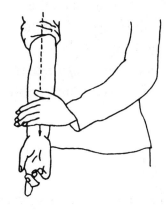

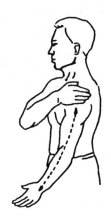

3. Rubbing the upper limbs: Rub with the palm of one hand along the medial side of the opposite upper limb from the armpit to the wrist and the lateral side of the limb from the wrist to the shoulder to and fro approximately 30 times on each side. Then rub the anterior, posterior, medial, and lateral aspects of the shoulder, the elbow, and the wrist until they feel warm.

4. Twisting the fingers: Hold each finger of each hand with the thumb and index finger of the other hand, twisting from the base of each finger to its tip several times for each finger.

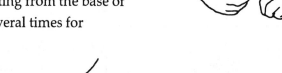

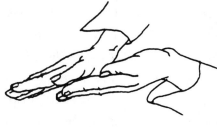

5. Rubbing the palms: Rub the palms against each other, beginning slowly and then speeding up until they get warm.

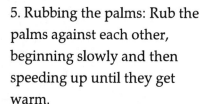

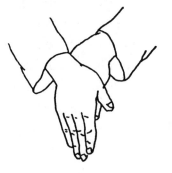

6. Rubbing the backs of the hands: Rub the back of one hand with the palm of the other hand starting slowly and then quickening the pace until it gets warm.

7. Grab emptiness with both hands: Stand erect with the feet shoulder-width apart. Raise the arms forward with the arms relaxed and the wrists flexed slightly backward as if one were grasping a large imaginary ball at the level of the chest. Then slightly flex and extend the fingers as if grasping onto something.

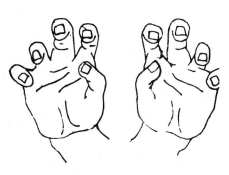

**Functions & indications:** These manipulations can be used for aches and pains in the upper limbs, periarthritis of the shoulder, tennis elbow, pain in wrists, numbness in fingers, etc. They relax the muscles of the upper limbs, relieve fatigue, improve the motor function of the upper limbs, and prevent motor and occupational injury.

## B. Self-massage of the lower limbs

**Massage methods:**

1. Pressing & kneading the points on the legs: Press and knead the following points with the tip of the thumb or the middle finger in the order of (1) *Ju Liao* (GB 29, located in the depression at the midpoint between the front spine of the pelvis and the head of the hip joint), (2) *Huan Tiao* (GB 30, located in the center of the buttock), *Fu Tu* (St 32, located 6

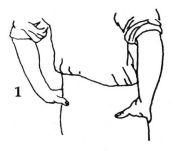

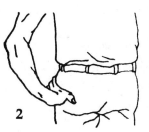

body inches above the lateral edge of the kneecap), (3) *Zu San Li* (St 36, located 3 body inches below the lateral side of the kneecap), (4) *Yang Ling Quan* (GB 34, located in the depression anterior and inferior to the small head of the fibula), (5) *Cheng Shan* (Bl 57, located in the center of the back of the calf at the top of the triangular angle where the two heads of the large muscle join), and (6) *San Yin Jiao* (Sp 6, located 3 body inches superior to the inner ankle). Press and knead each point 30-50 times.

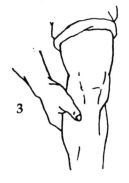
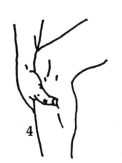
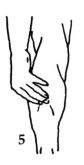
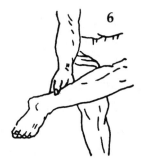

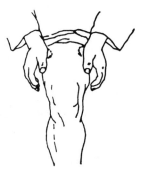

2. Pressing & kneading the thighs: Place both heels of the palms opposite to each other on the thigh. Press and knead the medial, lateral, anterior, and posterior sides of the thigh from top to bottom 3-5 times each side until there is a sensation of mild soreness and distention.

3. Pressing & kneading the kneecaps: Relax the leg. Grasp, pinch, press, and knead the kneecap with the thumb and the lateral surface of the index finger (which is bent like a bow) of one hand, producing a sensation of mild soreness and distention.

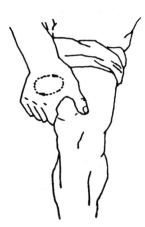

4. Grasping the shanks: Lift and grasp the muscles of the calf of the leg with the thumb, index, and middle fingers of one hand from the back of the knee to the heel with gentle force, producing a sensation of mild soreness and distention.

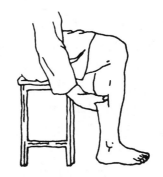

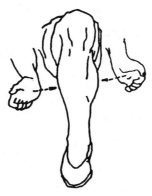

5. Patting the lower limbs: Pat the leg with both palms on opposite sides of the leg from the upper part of the thigh to the lower part of the lower leg approximately 20 times.

6. Rubbing *Yong Quan* (Ki 1): Rub rapidly and forcefully with the fleshy pad of muscle at the base of the little finger the sole of the opposite foot at *Yong Quan* (which is located in the depression just lateral to the ball of the foot) in order to produce a hot feeling.

7. Rotating the ankle joints: Sitting upright, hold the upper part of the ankle with one hand and the toes with the other hand. Rotate the ankle joint clockwise and counterclockwise approximately 20 times each ankle.

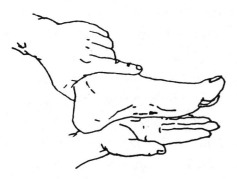

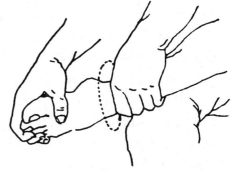

8. Press the leg & bend the waist: Standing upright, place the lower part of one leg on a stool. Put both hands on the knee. Then bend the waist and stretch the knee and press the leg several times. Switch legs and repeat this process on the other side.

**Functions & indications:** These manipulations can be used for soreness and pain of the lower limbs, lower limb sprains, swelling and pain in the joints and muscle spasms of the lower limbs. They relax the muscles, relieve fatigue, and improve the motor function of the lower limb joints. Therefore, they can be used for the health care of athletes and for preventing occupational injuries.

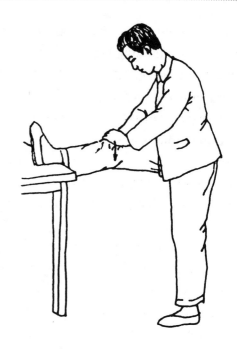

## Selecting the appropriate local self-massage manipulations

The repertoire of local self-massage manipulations introduced above have wide applications. They are the basis of Chinese self-massage for both the promotion of health and the treatment of disease. For general health care, these maneuvers can be done once or twice a day in the following order: the head and face, the neck and upper back, the upper limbs, the chest and abdomen, the lumbosacral region, and then the lower limbs. For those who work at professions which may easily cause local fatigue and repetitive strain, one should choose the appropriate manipulations for the affected areas of the body. For example, people who work day after day bending over desks often experience neck and upper back fatigue and tension. In that case, one should choose the self-massage manipulations for the neck, upper and lower backs. Athletes such as tennis players and weight-lifters who do a lot of upper limb exercises can benefit by self-massaging their upper limbs. People such as long distance runners and standing workmen should choose the self-massage routine for the lower limbs.

Local self-massage can also treat and prevent a variety of common diseases. For instance, pupils in primary or middle school who easily suffer from nearsightedness may perform self-massage of the face to relieve eyestrain. The middle-aged and the elderly who are easily affected by cervical spondylopathy can do self-massage on their neck, upper back, and upper limbs to prevent and treat cervical spondylopathy. Self-massage of the chest and the upper back can be done to prevent and treat asthma, bronchitis, and heart diseases. Self-massage of the abdomen and pressing and kneading on *Zu San Li* (St 36) on the lower limbs are effective for preventing and treating digestive system diseases, while self-massage on the head and rubbing *Yong Quan* (Ki 1) on the soles can prevent and treat hypertension.

Having chosen the appropriate location for local self-massage, one can lengthen or shorten the duration of the massage depending upon the time available and whether one is simply preventing disease or trying to treat disease and relieve localized fatigue and strain. In general, it is necessary to devote more time each session if one is trying to treat disease than to promote health and prevent disease.

Chinese self-massage manipulations should be done in a relaxed and light manner. In the beginning, the duration of the massage may be short. The time can then be gradually prolonged as one's skill in doing the manipulations also gradually develops. Self-massage for preventive health care can be done once every other day at the beginning, gradually increasing this to once every day.

# Chinese Self-massage for Beautification

Chinese self-massage for beautification of the face and body is mainly aimed at young and middle-aged people and especially women. Some women during puberty are vexed by acne. Many women develop liver spots and butterfly rashes on their faces during or after childbirth. For most women, as they age, their skin gradually becomes rough and wrinkled due to decline of endocrine function and the accumulated microtrauma of sun, wind, abrasion, and detergents.

Chinese self-massage for beautification consists of certain manipulations applied to the skin of the face and to acupuncture points on the body. Self-massage on the face improves the local circulation of blood and body fluids as well as the metabolism of the skin. Chinese self-massage manipulations stimulating certain acupuncture points on the body can help balance and revitalize the internal organs of the body, including the endocrine glands, excite the autonomic nerves, and adjust the relative equilibrium of the nerves and body fluids so as to improve the beauty of the face as well as the body as a whole.

## 1. Self-massage for moistening & nourishing the skin

In Chinese medicine, the moisture and luster of the skin is dependent on the qi and blood flow to the skin. In order for the skin to be moist and lustrous, the internal organs must transform and create sufficient blood to nourish the skin. On top of that, the qi and blood must be able to flow freely to and through the local areas, bringing the moistening blood and body fluids to nourish and repair the local tissue. The Chinese self-massage manipulations below are designed to stimulate the production of blood and to quicken the blood and move the qi through the local areas.

**Massage methods:**

1. Pressing & kneading the points on the face: Rinse the face with warm water and wipe it dry. Dip the fingers in an appropriate ointment to protect the skin depending on whether your skin is oily, medium, or dry. Then press and knead the points on the face on both sides in the following order: *Yang Bai* (GB 14, located on the forehead 1 body inch directly above the midpoint of the eyebrow), *Zan Zhu* (Bl 2, located in the depression at the medial edge of the eyebrow), *Jing Ming* (Bl 1, located 0.1 body inch medial and superior to the inner canthus of the eye), *Si Bai* (St 2, located in the depression directly below the center of the eye), *Tai Yang* (M-HN-9, located in the center of the temple, 1 body inch behind the lateral edge of the eyebrow and outer canthus), *Tong Zi Liao* (GB 1, located 0.5 body inch lateral to the outer canthus of the eye), *Si Zhu Kong* (TB 23, located at the lateral end of the eyebrow), *Yu Yao* (M-HN-6, located in the middle of the eyebrow), *Yin Tang* (M-HN-3, located midpoint between the eyebrows), *Xia Guan* (St 7, located at the lower border of the zygomatic arch in the depression in front of the condyloid process of the jaw), *Jia Che* (St 6, located one finger-width anterior and superior to the lower angle of the jaw), *Ying Xiang* (LI 20, located in the groove between the nose and the lips just lateral to the wings of the nose), and *Cheng Jiang* (CV 24, located in the depression in the center of the grove between the lower lip and the chin). Press and knead each point 30-50 times.

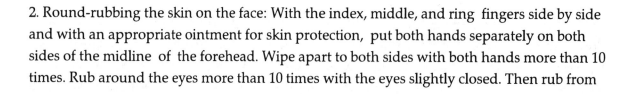

2. Round-rubbing the skin on the face: With the index, middle, and ring fingers side by side and with an appropriate ointment for skin protection, put both hands separately on both sides of the midline of the forehead. Wipe apart to both sides with both hands more than 10 times. Rub around the eyes more than 10 times with the eyes slightly closed. Then rub from

both sides of the nose to the corners of the mouth and, after that, along the lower sides of the cheeks and through the sides of the cheeks. Pass the corners of the eyes with slight force to the forehead and come at last back to the inner sides of the eyes and the sides of the nose. Rub the skin of the whole face in this circular way with light force more than 10 times until the face becomes moist and red. A suitable force will not make the skin fold.

3. Heating the face: Rub the palms against each other until they become hot. Then put them on both sides of the face and keep them on the face for 2-3 minutes.

4. Round-rubbing the abdomen: Rub around the abdomen in a circular manner and clockwise direction with the hollow of the palm for approximately 5 minutes.

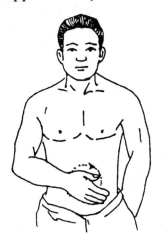

5. Pressing & kneading the points on the back: Press and knead with the knuckles of both thumbs the points 1.5 body inches lateral to both sides of the spine: *Gan Shu* (Bl 18, located at the level of the lower border of the 9th thoracic vertebra), *Pi Shu* (Bl 20,

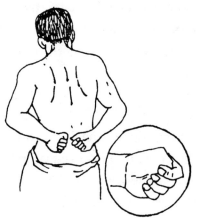

located lateral to the lower edge of the 11th thoracic vertebra), and *Shen Shu* (Bl 23, located lateral to the lower edge of the 2nd lumbar vertebra). Do this approximately 100 times each point. (Figure on previous page)

6. Lifting & pinching the skin of the back: Put both hands on the points on the sides of the spine described above. Pinch the skin on the points with the thumb, index, and middle fingers, lifting and releasing 3-5 times each point.

7. Straight rubbing the back: Place the palm on the governing vessels (*i.e.*, the midline of the back over the spine) and rub up and down this line until it feels hot. Then rub up and down the same way on the bladder channel located 1.5 body inches lateral to the midline.

8. Rubbing the lower limbs: Rub with the palm to and fro on the inner and outer sides of the thighs and shanks of both lower limbs until they feel warm.

9. Pressing & kneading *Zu San Li* (St 36): Press and knead with the thumb on the point 3 body inches below the lateral lower edge of the kneecap 30-50 times each leg.

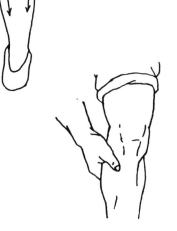

10. Pressing & kneading *Yong Quan* (Ki 1):
Press and knead with the thumb on the point
located in the depression lateral to the ball of
the foot at the junction between the front 1/3
and back 2/3 of the sole 30-50 times each foot.

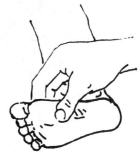

**Functions & indications:** These manipulations can
make the skin ruddy, glossy, and elastic and improve
the circulation of blood and lymph. They can be used for general
facial beautification. They are very effective for people whose skin is rough, pale, and dark.

## 2. Self-massage for preventing & treating acne

In Chinese medicine, acne is seen as the result of heat flaming upward in the body, over-
heating the blood in the face. Therefore, the Chinese self-massage of facial acne is designed
to eliminate pathological excess heat in the interior of the body. Mostly this heat accumulates
in the digestive tract. However, in adolescents in particular, this heat comes from the yang
energy of the kidneys which is suddenly maturing and stirring and causing maturation. In
addition, these self-massage maneuvers help dissipate any heat which has accumulated
locally in the face by stimulating and moving the qi and blood to and through these areas. If
the heat does not become stagnant and depressed locally, it will not form pimples.

**Massage methods:**

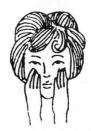

1. Rubbing the skin of the face: Wash the face and hands
clean with warm water. Put both hands gently on the
face and rub with a light force on the whole face
more than 10 times.

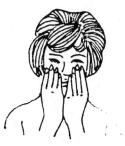

2. Heating the face: After heating the palms by rubbing them against each other, place them on both sides of the face and keep them on the face for 2-3 minutes.

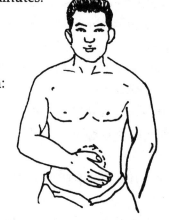

3. Round rubbing the abdomen: Round rub the abdomen around the navel clockwise with the hollow of the palm for approximately 5 minutes.

4. Pressing & kneading the points on the back: Press and knead with the knuckles of both thumbs the points 1.5 body inches lateral to both sides of the spine: *Pi Shu* (Bl 20, T 11), *Shen Shu* (Bl 23, L2), and *Da Chang Shu* (Bl 25, lateral to the lower edge of the 4th lumbar vertebra). Repeat this approximately 100 times on each point.

5. Straight rubbing the back: Place the palm on the governing vessel (*i.e.*, the midline of the spine) and rub straight up and down until there is a hot sensation. Then do this on the bladder channel 1.5 body inches lateral to the midline on each side of the spine.

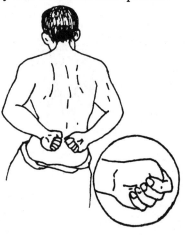

6. Finger striking & rubbing on the upper limbs: With the tips of the thumb, index, and middle fingers close to each other, strike on the three lines on the anterior, middle, and posterior line of the outside of the upper limb on the opposite side of the body. These three lines are the large intestine channel, the triple burner channel, and the small intestine channel. Strike from the wrist to the shoulder approximately 10 times each line. Then rub the outside of the limb from the wrist to the shoulder until hot. After finishing one side, repeat this procedure on the other side of the body.

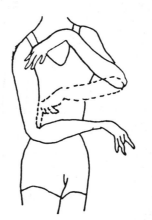
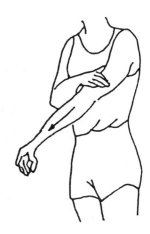

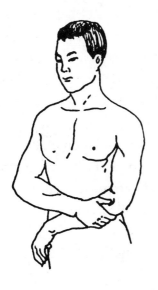

7. Pressing & kneading the points on the upper limbs: Press and knead with the thumb of one hand on the points of the opposite upper limb: *Jian Yu* (LI 15, located in the middle of the depression in the shoulder appearing when the arm is held straight out to the side just beyond the tip of the shoulder joint), *Qu Chi* (LI 11, located in the depression at the lateral end of the elbow crease when the elbow is flexed), and *He Gu* (LI 4, located in the center of the mound in the angle between the thumb and index finger). Press and knead each of these points 30-50 times. After finishing one side, repeat this procedure on the other side of the body.

41

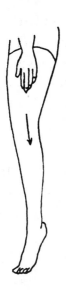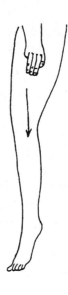

8. Finger-striking and rubbing on lower limbs: With the tips of the thumb, index, and middle fingers close to each other, strike on the line of the kidney channel on the back and inner side of the lower limb of the opposite side, starting from above and striking to below approximately 10 times. Then rub straight up and down this channel until hot. Strike and rub the other lower limb in the same way.

9. Pressing & kneading *Yong Quan* (Ki 1): Press and knead the point in the depression in the center of the sole just lateral to the ball of the foot 30-50 times. Do this on both feet.

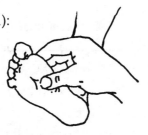

**Functions & indications:** These manipulations can improve the excretion of the sebaceous glands, remove inflammation caused by the blockage of the pores of the skin, and regulate the gastrointestinal functions and hormonal secretions. They can prevent and treat acne during puberty and acne caused by disorders of the gastrointestinal function.

## 3. Self-massage for protecting & securing the teeth

In Chinese medicine, the teeth are seen as the surplus or outgrowth of the bones and the bones are the tissue associated with the Chinese medical concept of the kidneys. The teeth are healthy and secure when the kidney qi is full and sufficient. Therefore, the self-massage manipulations described below help to supplement the kidneys. In addition, the qi and blood in the local areas of the teeth must also be freely flowing and not stagnant or depressed. Other of the self-massage manipulations given below help insure that the qi and blood flowing to and nourishing and empowering the teeth is smoothly and freely flowing.

**Massage methods:**

1. Clicking the teeth: Click the upper and lower teeth against each other 30-50 times. The force should be slight at the beginning and should gradually increase. The number of clicks should also be gradually increased. Do this once in the morning and once in the evening or several times per day.

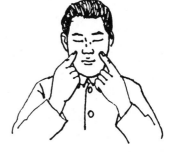

2. Pressing & kneading *Xia Guan* (St 7) and *Jia Che* (St 6): Press and knead with both middle fingers on the points *Xia Guan* (located in the depression below the zygomatic arch in front of the mandibular joint) and *Jia Che* (located anterior and superior to the angle of the jaw) approximately 100 times each.

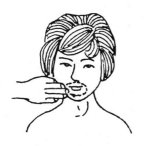

3. Circular rubbing the lips: Hold the index, middle, and ring fingers of one hand side by side. Then rub them around the lips at the level of the gums with slight force 5-10 times.

4. Pressing & kneading *He Gu* (LI 4): Press and knead *He Gu* which is located in the middle of the bulge in the angle between the thumb and index finger. Pressing with the thumb of one hand on the point of the other hand approximately 100 times on each side.

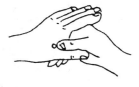

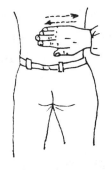

5. Transverse rubbing the lumbosacral area: Rub with one palm transversely to and fro on the lumbosacral area until a hot feeling penetrates inside the body.

**Functions & indications:** These manipulations can be used for preventing and treating tooth diseases. They can strengthen the teeth and are mainly used for prevention. However, they can also be used for treating loose teeth, toothache, receding gums, and bleeding gums.

# 4. Self-massage for protecting & securing the hair

In Chinese medicine, the hair is seen as the surplus or outgrowth of the blood and blood is part of the body's overall yin fluids. Therefore, the self-massage manipulations in this section either promote the production and replenishment of yin, blood, and body fluids so that these can then moisten and nourish the hair, or they stimulate the flow of qi and blood in the local area.

**Massage methods:**

1. Scrubbing & kneading the skin of the head: Scrub and knead with one palm on the whole head laying emphasis on any area of hair loss. The manipulation should be light but maintained until it feels hot in the local area.

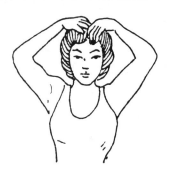

2. Combing the skin of the head: Comb the hair with the four fingers of one hand on the top and same side of the head from front to back and then comb the other side with the other hand 30-50 times altogether. The four fingers should scrape on the scalp while combing, and the force should not be too strong.

3. Patting the crown of the head: Pat all over the top part of the head lightly with one empty palm 30-50 times.

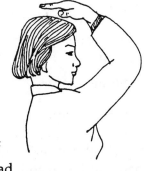

4. Five fingers grasping the crown of the head: Grasp the crown of the head with the five fingers of one hand from the anterior hairline to the posterior hairline 10-20 times. The middle finger should be in the middle and the other four fingers should be held apart naturally. The middle finger should grasp the midline of the head, while the other fingers should grasp both sides. The grasping movement should be quick, even, and gentle.

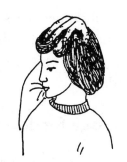

5. Rubbing the inner sides of the legs: Rub the inner sides of the shank and thigh from bottom to top and from the inner ankle to the knee with one palm several times. Then rub from the inner side of the knee to the base of the thigh several times until a hot sensation is produced.

6. Pressing & kneading *San Yin Jiao* (Sp 6): Press and knead the point 3 body inches above the tip of the inner ankle on the posterior border of the medial aspect of the tibia 30-50 times on each leg.

7. Rubbing *Yong Quan* (Ki 1): With the fleshy pad of muscle at the base of each little finger, rapidly and forcefully rub the depression lateral to the ball of the foot on the sole of the opposite side until a hot feeling is produced.

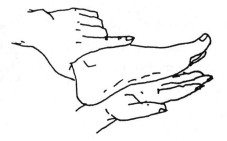

**Functions & indications:** These manipulations improve the blood circulation of the scalp and thus the nourishment of the hair follicles. In addition, they adjust the nervous system. Therefore they are effective for making the hair shiny and lustrous and for preventing and treating dandruff.

# 5. Self-massage for developing the breasts

In Chinese medicine, the muscles and flesh are created out of the qi and blood which nourish them. Therefore, the self-massage maneuvers and exercises below are all designed to promote maximum flow of qi and blood to and through the area of the breasts. Likewise, it is the qi which holds up and in or tones the body tissues. If there is sufficient qi in an area, then the tissue in that area will tend to be firm and not sag or droop.

**Massage methods:**

1. Pressing & kneading *Ru Gen* (St 18): Press and knead with both middle fingers separately on *Ru Gen* (located 1 body inch below both nipples) approximately 100 times until there is a slight sore sensation.

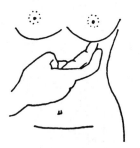

2. Pushing the breasts: Place one palm on each breast and push each breast from superior, inferior, medial, and lateral directions towards the nipples approximately 10 times in each direction. This pushing should be slow, deep, and forceful.

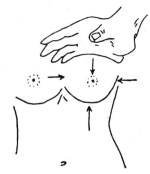

3. Kneading & circular rubbing the breasts: Place one palm on each breast. Then knead and circular rub the breasts for 2-3 minutes. The force should go from weak to strong as the rubbing continues.

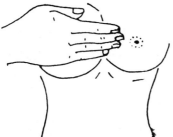

4. Vibrating & pushing the breasts: Cup the breasts in the palms. Then push them upward while vibrating the palms, moving from the lower edge of the breasts to the nipples 5-10 times. The vibration should be quick but the pushing should be slow.

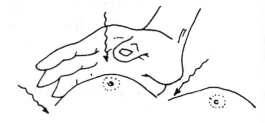

5. Pushing & squeezing the breasts: Place the two palms on the sides of one of the breasts. There should be a wide angle between the thumbs and fingers. Then push and squeeze the breast by drawing the thumb and index finger together. Push and squeeze the breasts to the nipples approximately 30-50 times for each breast. Then hold both nipples with the fingers of both hands, kneading and twisting them while slightly pulling on them at the same time 5-10 times.

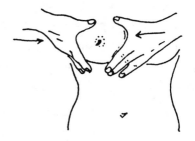

6. Upper limb movement: To do this maneuver, one may either sit or stand erect. Extend the arms straight out in front with the palms facing each other and arms parallel to the ground. Move the arms out to the sides, expanding the chest, 30-50 times. Then raise the arms over the head another 30-50 times.

7. Push-ups: Do push-ups 15-20 times each time, 3 times per day.

8. Weight-lifting: While lying on one's back, do bench presses with a suitable amount of weight so that one can just do 15-20 repetitions. Then, standing erect with feet shoulder-width apart, use hand weights in each hand. Alternately lift one hand weight across the chest to the front of the opposite shoulder. Then do this with the weight in the other hand. Do 15-20 repetitions on each side, 3 times per day.

**Functions & indications:** These manipulations can help adjust the secretion of hormones and improve the growth of the breasts. They can be used for enlarging small breasts which are undeveloped and also for toning inelastic and flat chests.

# 6. Self-massage for losing weight

Adipose tissue or fat in Chinese medicine is seen as an accumulation of phlegm and dampness. Therefore, if one wants to keep the accumulation of phlegm and dampness from becoming excessive, then one should make sure that the viscera responsible for creating phlegm and dampness when they underfunction are kept in tip-top shape. The two viscera which are responsible in Chinese medicine for the creation and transformation of body fluids and, therefore, phlegm and dampness are the spleen and kidneys. Therefore, the self-massage manipulations given in this section help insure that the spleen and kidneys are functioning correctly. Since the spleen in Chinese medicine stands for the process of digestion, these self-massage maneuvers also insure proper stomach and intestinal function. If the spleen and kidneys function the way they should, then their yang qi or energy will melt or burn away fat automatically.

**Massage methods:**

1. Circular rubbing the abdomen: Rub with the palm of the hand circularly around the navel clockwise approximately 5-10 minutes. The force should be slightly strong and speed should be a little bit fast.

2. Pressing & kneading *Pi Shu* (Bl 20) and *Shen Shu* (Bl 23): Press and knead with the knuckles of the thumbs on the paired points *Pi Shu* (located 1.5 body inches lateral to the lower edge of the 11th thoracic vertebra) and *Shen Shu* (located 1.5 body inches lateral to the lower edge of the 2nd lumbar vertebra) approximately 100 times each. The force should be heavy in order to produce a strong sensation of soreness and distention.

3. Straight-rubbing the back: Rub with the side of the hand on the governing vessel in the midline of the back directly over the spine. Then rub the bladder channel located 1.5 body inches lateral to the spine. Rub up and down to produce a hot sensation.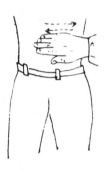

4. Transverse rubbing the lumbosacral region: Rub transversely back and forth across the lumbosacral region with the palm of the hand to produce a hot sensation.

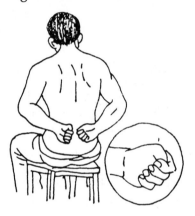

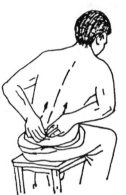

5. Rubbing the medial sides of the lower limbs: With each palm, alternately rub the medial side of the opposite leg from the base of the thigh to the knee 5-10 times and then from the knee to the inner ankle 5-10 times in order to produce a hot sensation.

6. Finger pressing *Cheng Fu* (Bl 36): With the knuckles of the bent thumbs, press *Cheng Fu* (located in the center of the fold of the buttocks at the top of each leg) approximately 100 times each to produce a sensation of mild soreness and distention.

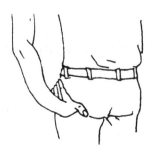

49

7. Pressing & kneading *Xue Hai* (Sp 10) and *Liang Qiu* (St 34): With each thumb, press and knead *Xue Hai* (located 2 body inches superior and medial to the upper, inner edge of the kneecap) and *Liang Qiu* (2 body inches superior and lateral to the upper, outer edge of the kneecap) approximately 100 times each point per leg until there is a mild sensation of soreness and distention.

8. Raising the legs when lying on one's back: Begin by lying on the back. Breathe in while slowly raising both legs by flexing from the hips. Raise the legs to a 90° angle. Then breathe out while slowly lowering the legs back down to the floor. Repeat this approximately 10 times. This exercise is best done on an empty stomach.

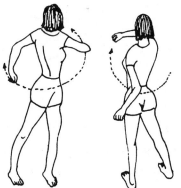

9. Swing the arms & turn the waist: Standing erect with feet shoulder-width apart, turn the waist to the right and to the left as far as one can rotate. While rotating, swing the arms beside the body simultaneously in coordination with the movement of the waist. Do this movement approximately 10 times.

**Functions & indications:** These manipulations and exercises are effective for burning fat, improving the metabolism, and regulating the functions of the kidneys, spleen, and stomach. They can be used for reducing body weight and keeping the body vigorous and graceful.

# 7. Self-massage for gaining weight & strengthening the body

As mentioned above, the muscles and flesh are created out of the nourishment supplied by the qi and blood. Therefore, for persons who are underweight, the emphasis in Chinese medicine is to supplement and regulate those viscera and bowels which play a part in the creation and circulation of the qi and blood. These viscera and bowels begin with the stomach and intestines, including the spleen, and also include the Chinese ideas of the liver and kidneys. Therefore, the self-massage techniques given below all supplement and regulate these viscera and bowels and insure the smooth and free flow of the qi and blood throughout the body so that it can nourish and construct the muscles and flesh.

**Massage methods:**

1. Circular rubbing the abdomen: Rub with the palm of the hand around the navel clockwise slowly with a gentle force for approximately 10 minutes. If one often has diarrhea, loose stools after each meal, abdominal bloating after meals, or undigested food in the stools, rub the abdomen counterclockwise.

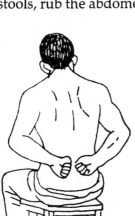

2. Pressing & kneading the points on the back: With the knuckles of the bent thumbs, press and knead the paired points at the sides of the spine in the following order: *Gan Shu* (Bl 18, located 1.5 body inches lateral to the lower edge of the 9th thoracic vertebra), *Pi Shu* (Bl 20, located 1.5 body inches lateral to the lower edge of the 11th thoracic vertebra), *Wei Shu* (Bl 21, located 1.5 body inches lateral to the lower edge of the 12th thoracic vertebra), and *Shen Shu* (Bl 23, located 1.5 body inches lateral to the lower edge of the 2nd lumbar vertebra) approximately 100 times each until there is a mild sensation of soreness and distention.

51

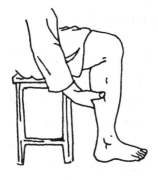

3. Grasping the lower limbs: With the thumb and the other four fingers of each hand, separately grasp and lift the muscles on the back side of each leg from the hip to the heel approximately 10 times. Then repeat this procedure on the front side of each leg from the base of the thigh to the ankle again approximately 10 times. The force of grasping should be gentle and deep. The movement down the leg should be done by grasping, releasing, and then moving downward the width of the hand.

4. Pressing & kneading *Xue Hai* (Sp 10) and *Zu San Li* (St 36): With each thumb, press and knead *Xue Hai* (located 2 body inches superior and medial to the upper, inside edge of the kneecap) and *Zu San Li* (located 3 body inches inferior and lateral to the outside, lower edge of the kneecap) on each leg approximately 100 times each point.

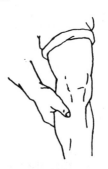

5. Pinching & pulling the spine: This manipulation should be done by a family member or friend. It cannot be done by oneself. First, apply some massage media to the back. Then, lightly massage along the middle of the spine from top to bottom 3-5 times. Next, place the hands on each side of the tailbone and grasp and lift the skin with the thumbs and the index and middle fingers of both hands, rolling the skin upward from the tailbone to the base of the neck approximately 10 times.

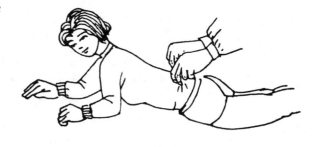

**Functions & indications:** These manipulations can be used by those whose body's are thin and weak in order to improve their health and bodily constitution. This is because these manipulations regulate the gastrointestinal functions of digestion and absorption, strengthen the appetite and the constitution, regulate the internal secretions, and thus improve the storage of fat.

# Chinese Self-massage for Improving Sexual Function

Chinese self-massage for improving sexual function is aimed at correcting certain factors and diseases which affect one's sexual life or make one's sexual life uncoordinated with their partner's. It can remove sexual dysfunction, enhance sexual function, and make the sex life of two partners happy and harmonious. There are lots of factors which can affect sexual life. Some of these affect the male, while others affect the female. Some of these factors may be pathological, some may be physiological, and some may be psychological. When there are problems with sexual function, some people are too embarrassed to see a doctor to discuss the matter and undergo examination. However, sexual function disorders can affect the physical and emotional relationship between two partners. Thus sexual function problems can place a mental and emotional burden on those who experience these. Happily, Chinese self-massage methods for correcting these problems are simple, painless, and free and can be self-administered or mutually administered between two partners. The manipulations below can regulate sexual function in order to preserve health and happiness and treat sexual function diseases remedially.

## 1. Self-massage for enhancing sexual desire

In Chinese medicine, sexual desire or libido is seen as the expression of the fire of life associated with the yang energy of the kidneys. In women, this yang energy tends to decrease beginning at around 35 years of age and in men at around 48. When diminished sexual desire is due to the natural effects of aging, the following Chinese self-massage manipulations may help restore the yang energy and function of the kidneys and fire of life.

**Massage methods:**

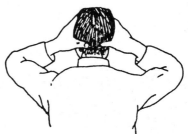

1. Pressing & kneading *Yi Feng* (TB 17) and *Feng Chi* (GB 20): With the middle fingers of both hands, press and knead *Yi Feng* (located behind the lower edge of the earlobe and below and in front of the bulging bone behind the ear) and *Feng Chi* (located behind the bulging bone behind the ear and 1 body inch above the hairline) on both sides approximately 100 times each until there is a sensation of mild soreness and distention.

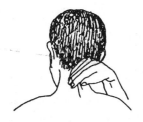

2. Grasping the muscles on the sides of the nape: With the thumb and the index and middle fingers opposing each other, grasp at the sides of the nape of the neck from the posterior hairline to the base of the neck approximately 10 times.

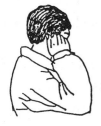

3. Twisting the helices: Pinch the helices of both ears gently with the thumbs and the lateral sides of the index fingers, twisting and rubbing up and down repeatedly approximately 10 times. Then hold the earlobes, pulling with gentle force 3-5 times.

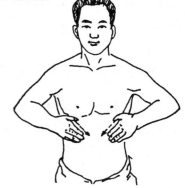

4. Rubbing the lateral costal region: Place the two palms against the region under the armpits and rub up and down to the level of the navel more than 10 times. Then rub to and fro from the armpits to the midline of the abdomen more than 10 times to produce a hot sensation.

54

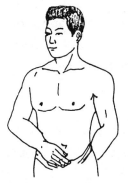

5. Pressing & kneading the points on the lower abdomen: With the middle finger of one hand, press and knead *Qi Hai* (CV 6, located 1.5 body inches below the navel), *Guan Yuan* (CV 4, located 3 body inches below the navel), *Zhong Ji* (CV 3, located 4 body inches below the navel), and *Qu Gu* (CV 2, located at the midpoint of the upper border of the pubic bone) approximately 100 times each point.

6. Pressing & kneading the points on the back: With the knuckles of the bent thumbs, press and knead the paired points at the sides of the spine in the following order: *Xin Shu* (Bl 15, located 1.5 body inches lateral to the 5th thoracic vertebra), *Ge Shu* (Bl 17, located 1.5 body inches lateral to the 7th thoracic vertebra), *Gan Shu* (Bl 18, located 1.5 body inches lateral to the 9th thoracic vertebra), and *Shen Shu* (Bl 23, located 1.5 body inches lateral to the 2nd lumbar vertebra) approximately 100 times each to produce a sensation of mild soreness and distention.

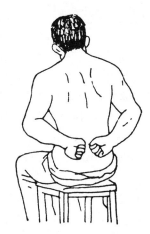

7. Transverse rubbing of the lumbosacral area: With one palm, rub transversely back and forth across the lumbosacral area to produce a sensation of heat. (See page 49, #4)

8. Pressing & kneading *Chang Qiang* (GV 1) and *Hui Yin* (CV 1): With the middle finger, press and knead *Chang Qiang* (located 0.5 body inches below the tip of tailbone) and *Hui Yin* (located at the midpoint between the vagina and the anus in a woman or the scrotum and anus in a man) approximately 200 times each point until there is a sensation of mild soreness and distention.

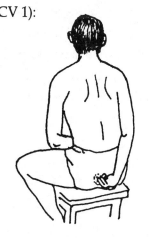

9. Twisting & kneading the genitalia: With the thumb and other fingers in opposition, gently twist and knead the genitals. In males, first twist and knead the scrotum and then the penis for approximately 2 minutes. In females, gently twist and knead the labia majora and surrounding region approximately 2 minutes.

10. Rubbing the medial sides (insides) of the thighs: With the left palm, rub the inner side of the right thigh up and down to produce a sensation of heat. Repeat this on the other thigh with the right palm.

11. Rubbing *Yong Quan* (Ki 1): With the fleshy pad of muscle at the base of the little finger, rub rapidly and forcefully on the sole of the opposite foot the point *Yong Quan* (located lateral to the ball of the foot) in order to produce a hot sensation.

**Functions & indications:** These manipulations can regulate the internal functions of the body, enhance sexual desire, supplement the kidneys, strengthen the waist, and strengthen the constitution. They are good for either males or females with no or low sexual desire, inability to ejaculate or orgasm, or sexual inhibition.

Chinese self-massage for increasing sexual desire should be done once a day, before going to bed in the evening. Chinese herbal medicine is also very effective for restoring and increasing sexual desire. However, Chinese herbs which supplement the yang energy of the kidneys should not be used as aphrodisiacs unnecessarily or for prolonged periods of time as they may cause problems. Chinese self-massage for increasing the libido has no side effects and only results in better health and function.

## 2. Impotence

Impotence refers to a man's inability to attain or maintain a hard enough erection so as to successfully perform sexual intercourse. In Chinese medicine, there are a number of causes of impotence. The following self-massage manipulations primarily treat impotence due to the natural weakening of the kidneys and fire of life with aging. Such self-massage can slow down this decline and, in fact, restore and supplement the yang energy of the kidneys.

**Massage methods:**

1. Pressing & kneading *Shen Que* (CV 8) and *Guan Yuan* (CV 4): With the thumb or middle finger of one hand, press and knead *Shen Que* (the navel) and *Guan Yuan* ( located 3 body inches below the navel) approximately 100 times each. Then, knead the area of *Guan Yuan* (*i.e.*, the middle of the lower abdomen) with the palm of the hand approximately 100 times.

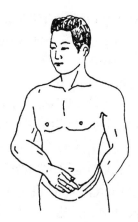

2.Pressing & kneading the genital area: With the tip of the middle finger, press and knead *Qu Gu* (CV 2, located at the midpoint of the superior edge of the pubic bone) and above and the sides of the root of the penis approximately 100 times each point. The force of kneading should gradually increase from weak to strong.

3. Twisting & kneading the penis: With the index and middle fingers of both hands holding the penis, lightly twist the penis, moving from the root to the glans of the penis. Then hold the glans and pull it several times, twisting, kneading, and pulling like this approximately 10 times. The force should be gentle.

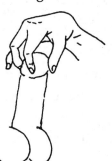

4. Twisting & kneading the scrotum: With the two palms, hold the scrotum and press it lightly in opposite directions approximately 50 times. The force goes from weak to strong to produce a sensation of mild soreness and distention. Then lightly twist and knead the scrotum approximately 100 times.

5. Finger pressing *Hui Yin* (CV 1): With the tip of the middle finger, press *Hui Yin* (the midpoint between the scrotum and the anus) approximately 100 times. (See page 55, bottom)

6. Pressing & kneading the points on the lower back: With the two thumbs, press and knead the paired points *Shen Shu* (Bl 23, located 1.5 body inches lateral to the lower border of the spinous process of the 2nd lumbar vertebra). Then with one thumb, press and knead *Ming Men* (GV 4, just below the spinous process of the 2nd lumbar vertebra) and *Yao Yang Guan* (GV 3, just below the spinous process of the 4th lumbar vertebra) 100-200 times each.

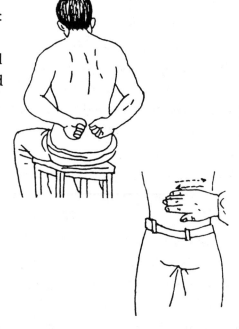

7. Transversely rubbing the lumbosacral area: With the palm of one hand, transversely rub the lumbosacral region to produce a hot sensation.

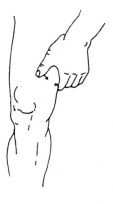

8. Grasping & kneading the thighs: First, with the thumb and other four fingers in opposition, grasp the inner and back sides from the base of the thigh to the knee for approximately 2 minutes. Then, with the palm, press and knead the inner and back sides of the thigh another 2 minutes. Lastly, pat the inner and back sides of the thigh 3-5 times each side. Then grasp and knead the other thigh in the same way.

**Functions & indications:** These manipulations can strengthen the body and sexual function. They can be used to improve male sexual function in general and for the treatment of impotence with either lack of penile erection, incomplete penile erection, or inability to maintain an erection during sexual intercourse.

Chinese self-massage for impotence should be done once a day before going to bed. Sexual intercourse should be avoided during the course of treatment. This is in order to allow the treatment to attain a cumulative effect. If one has sex too soon after starting this treatment, its affects will be squandered prematurely.

# 3. Premature ejaculation

Premature ejaculation refers to uncontrollable and unwanted ejaculation. This may occur before the insertion of the penis, during the insertion of the penis, or anytime before the partner orgasms and the individual chooses to ejaculate. Although there are several different causes of premature ejaculation in Chinese medicine, many cases are due to insufficient kidney yin energy. This is just the opposite of the yang deficiency described above under impotence. Here the fire of life becomes too inflamed and excited too quickly and so it loses control over the yin semen which then slips out uncontrollably. Hence the following self-massage manipulations are primarily aimed at supplementing and nourishing the yin energy of the kidneys so that it may keep the yang energy in sufficient check.

**Massage methods:**

1. Circular rubbing the abdomen: With the center of one palm, rub around the navel counterclockwise for approximately 5 minutes.

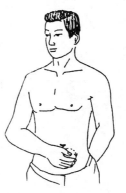

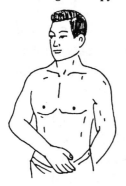

2. Pressing & kneading *Guan Yuan* (CV 4): With the thumb or the middle finger, press and knead *Guan Yuan* (located 3 body inches below the navel) approximately 100 times. There will be better results if a local sensation of soreness and distention spreading to the penis is produced.

3. Striking the lumbosacral area & buttocks: Make fists with both hands. With the back of each fist, alternately strike the lumbosacral area and buttocks for approximately 2 minutes. The degree of force is correct if a vibrating and comfortable feeling is produced in the local area.

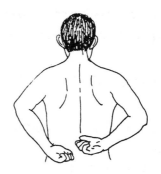

4. Pressing & kneading *Zu San Li* (St 36) and *San Yin Jiao* (Sp 6): With the tip of each thumb separately press and knead *Zu San Li* (located 3 body inches below and to the side of the inferior, lateral border of the kneecap) and *San Yin Jiao* (located 3 body inches above the tip of the inner ankle) approximately 100 times each point on each leg until there is a sensation of mild soreness and distention.

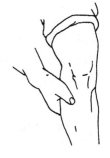

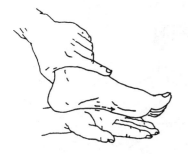

5. Rubbing *Yong Quan* (Ki 1): With the fleshy pad of muscle at the base of the little finger, rub the sole of the opposite foot at the point *Yong Quan* (located in the depression lateral to the ball of the foot) to produce a hot feeling.

6. Squeezing & pressing the penis: In the course of sexual intercourse, hold the glans penis with the thumb and index and middle fingers in opposition and squeeze and press it for 4-5 seconds. Then release suddenly. Squeeze and press like this once every several minutes during the whole course of sexual intercourse.

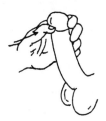

7. Squeezing & pressing the root of the penis: This manipulation may be done after the symptom of premature ejaculation has improved. Squeeze and press the root of the penis with the thumb and index and middle fingers during the course of sexual intercourse. The manipulation method is the same as squeezing & pressing the penis above.

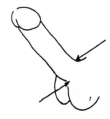

**Functions & indications:** These manipulations strengthen sexual function and control nocturnal emission. They can be used for the treatment of loss of erection prematurely during intercourse and premature ejaculation during intercourse. They can also relieve the concomitant symptoms of vertigo, listlessness, insomnia, and dream-disturbed sleep as well as lassitude in loins and legs due to premature ejaculation.

Manipulations 1-5 should be done once a day, and one month equals one course of treatment. Treatment should generally be done for 3-4 courses. Manipulations 6 & 7 are done during sexual intercourse itself.

## 4. Chronic prostatitis & benign prostatic hypertrophy

Chronic prostatitis is a common male urological disease in middle-aged adults. Chronic prostatitis mainly manifests as pain in the lower abdomen, low back pain, discomfort and soreness in the perineum and testes, increase of urethral secretion, possible frequent urination, urgency to urinate, and a burning, astringent sensation in the urethra when urinating. There may also be pain during ejaculation, premature ejaculation, and blood in the semen. Therefore, chronic prostatitis may affect one's sexual enjoyment and function. In severe cases, the patient's fertility may be affected.

Benign prostatic hypertrophy refers to nonmalignant swelling and hardening of the prostate. This is a common condition in older middle-aged and elderly men. Its symptoms are perineal soreness especially when sitting for a long time, frequent urge to urinate but either a weak stream or incomplete evacuation, terminal dribbling, and frequent and repeated nocturnal urination due to inability to completely empty the bladder. If this condition becomes severe, it may lead to complete cessation of urination requiring catheterization and/or surgery.

**Massage methods:**

1. Circular rubbing the *Dan Tian:* Circularly rub the area of the midpoint of the lower abdomen with one palm clockwise for approximately 5 minutes.

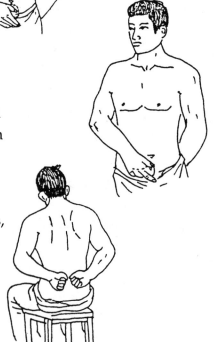

2. Finger pressing *Zhong Ji* (CV 3): With the tip of one middle finger, press *Zhong Ji* (located 4 body inches below the navel). First, press with force gradually deeper and deeper. Then turn the tip of the finger in the direction of the perineum and keep pressing about 30 seconds. Then suddenly relax. Do this 5-10 times. One should create a feeling of mild soreness and distention in the local area.

3. Pressing & kneading *Shen Shu* (Bl 23): With both thumbs, press and knead the paired points *Shen Shu* (located 1.5 body inches lateral to the lower border of the 2nd lumbar vertebra) 100-200 times. One should produce a sensation of mild soreness and distention in the local area.

4. Transversely rubbing the lumbosacral region: Rub the lumbosacral region to and fro with one palm to produce a sensation of heat. Best results will be achieved if the sensation of heat is felt all the way in the abdomen. (See picture, page 58, #7)

5. Rubbing and kneading the medial side of the thigh: With each palm, press and knead the inner side of each thigh. Then rub up and down along the inner side of each thigh alternately to produce a sensation of heat.

6. Pressing & kneading *San Yin Jiao* (Sp 6), *Tai Xi* (Ki 3), and *Tai Chong* (Liv 3): With both thumbs, press and knead the paired points on both legs beginning with (1) *San Yin Jiao* (located 3 body inches above the tip of the inner ankle). Next press and knead (2) *Tai Xi* (located at the midpoint between the inner ankle and the Achilles tendon). Then press and knead (3) *Tai Chong* (located on the back of the foot in the depression just in front of the junction of the 1st and 2nd metatarsal bones). Repeat these manipulations approximately 100 times for each point.

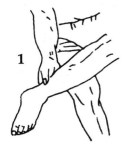
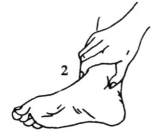
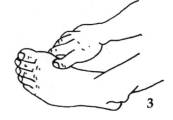

7. Rotating the hip joints: Lie on the back, flex the hip and the knee of one leg, and rotate each hip joint one at a time for approximately 1 minute each.

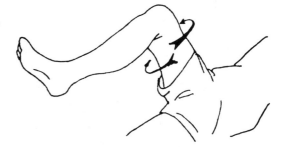

8. Pressing & kneading the prostate: Wearing a latex examination glove, first lightly rub around the anus with the index, middle, and ring fingers of one hand. Then slowly insert the middle finger into the anus and press the anterior wall of the anus. When touching the prostate, you may feel a little hard lump under the tip of the finger. Lightly press and knead this lump approximately 100 times. After withdrawing the middle finger from the anus, press and knead the perineum between the anus and the testes approximately 100 times.

**Functions & indications:** These manipulations quicken the blood and supplement the kidneys, scatter nodulation and soften hardness. They can help in the treatment and prevention of both chronic prostatitis and benign prostatic hypertrophy.

For the treatment of acute prostatitis, one should use antibiotics and/or acupuncture and Chinese herbal medicine. For the treatment of chronic prostatitis and benign prostatic hypertrophy, Chinese self-massage can be a very effective adjunctive treatment when combined with acupuncture and/or Chinese herbal medicine. These diseases' course is quite long and they also easily relapse. Therefore, persons with either of these diseases should persist in their self-massage and general health preservation. In the case of chronic prostatitis, it is important to avoid spicy, hot, peppery food and alcohol. In both conditions, it is important to keep the bowels open and freely flowing.

CHAPTER
5

# Chinese Self-massage for Treating Common Diseases

As mentioned in the Introduction, all disease in Chinese medicine is seen as imbalance. Either the viscera and bowels are over- or under-functioning or the qi and/or blood are not flowing freely and smoothly through a certain area. Because the entire body is connected into one unified whole by the system of channels and network vessels, stimulating certain areas of the body through self-massage can stimulate the flow of qi and blood and, therefore, also stimulate and regulate the function of the internal organs. When the qi and blood flow freely and without obstruction and the viscera and bowels all function up to par and in a harmonious and concerted way, then disease is cured and health is restored. Thus Chinese self-massage can most definitely be used to treat and cure a wide variety of common diseases.

In fact, Chinese self-massage can be used to treat diseases in all the specialty departments of Chinese medicine: internal medicine, external medicine, gynecology, traumatology, and diseases of the five sense organs. For some diseases, Chinese self-massage can be used as the sole or main treatment, while in others it functions as a supporting or adjunctive treatment, supplementing and extending the effects of other treatment modalities, Eastern or Western.

Professional practitioners of traditional Chinese medicine have their own system of diagnosis in which they identify many different patterns under a single disease. Since people vary as to their age, sex, physique, diet, occupation, and so many other factors, two people with the same disease still typically present a different pattern of signs and symptoms if one takes into account all their body functions. It is diagnosis and treatment based on the total pattern of signs and symptoms of a patient which makes traditional Chinese medicine the holistic medicine it is. It does not just treat diseases but treats the entire patient as a unique pattern of expression.

However, learning to do a professional Chinese medical pattern discrimination or diagnosis takes several years of intensive study and is beyond the scope of a layperson's guide such as this. Happily, because different diseases do share common important disease mechanisms and symptoms, one can identify the main mechanisms at work in each disease and can address these main mechanisms with Chinese self-massage. However, if Chinese self-massage fails to achieve an adequate or timely effect, readers should see a professional medical practitioner, be that a Western MD or an acupuncturist or practitioner of Chinese medicine.

# 1. Self-massage for internal medicine diseases

## A. Common cold

The common cold or flu is a common, infectious, upper respiratory disease usually due to viral contagion. Its main symptoms are headache, stuffy nose, runny nose, sneezing, chills, and fever. It may occur in any season but is most common in the winter and spring. Although colds tend to run a certain course, Chinese self-massage is very effective for relieving the discomfort of their initial stages and for preventing the cold from going deeper into the body where it may cause bronchitis or some other upper respiratory disease.

In Chinese medicine, the common cold is described as an invasion of the superficial layer or exterior of the body by evil wind. This wind, meaning an unseen pathogen, enters the upper body through certain acupuncture points called wind gates and then interferes with the flow of qi and blood through the exterior of the body and with the function of the lungs. Thus Chinese self-massage maneuvers for treating the symptoms of the common cold are aimed at stimulating the wind points, moving the qi and blood in the exterior of the body, and regulating and restoring the function of the lungs.

**Massage methods:**

1. Opening heaven's gate: Push upward along the midline of the forehead from the midpoint between the eyebrows to the anterior hairline with the index and middle fingers of both hands. Begin at the level of the eyebrows and alternately push upward to the hairline again and again, 50-100 times, pushing in one direction only, from the eyebrows upward to the hairline.

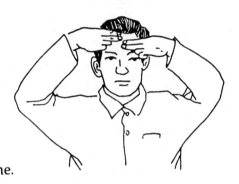

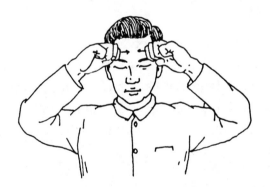

2. Pushing apart on the forehead: Bend the two index fingers and push with the lateral sides of their middle segments from the midline of the forehead to the anterior hairline on both sides of the forehead and the ends of the eyebrows. Do this approximately 100 times.

3. Kneading *Tai Yang* (M-HN- 9): Press with the tip of the thumbs or middle fingers on the points *Tai Yang* located 1 body inch lateral to the lateral end of each eyebrow and outer corner of the eye and knead them approximately 100 times until there is a sensation of mild soreness and distention.

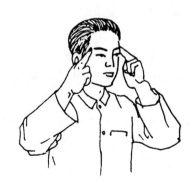

67

4. Wiping the temples: Press the temples with the pads of the thumbs and wipe backwards repeatedly with force approximately 100 times until there is a sensation of mild soreness and distention.

5. Pressing & kneading *Feng Chi* (GB 20): With the tips of both thumbs, press and knead the paired points *Feng Chi* (located in the depression between the upper portion of the sternocleidomastoid muscle and trapezius, 1 body inch within the hairline) approximately 100 times. The force should be strong enough to make the forehead sweat.

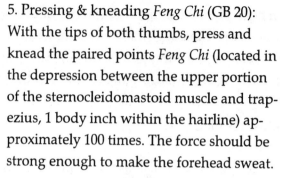

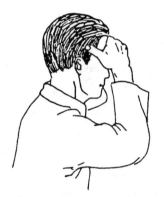

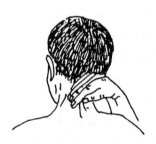

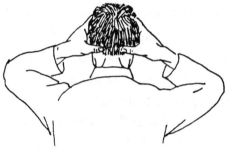

6. Grasping the muscles on both sides of the nape: Put the thumb of one hand on one side of the nape and the index and middle fingers on the other side, grasping the muscles of both sides from the posterior hairline to the base of the neck 10-20 times.

7. Grasping & pounding *Jian Jing* (GB 21): With the thumb, index, and middle fingers of the left hand, grasp the right *Jian Jing* (located at the midpoint of the top of the shoulder) 3-5 times. Then switch hands and grasp the left *Jian Jiang* with the right hand. Next, pound the point with an empty fist 30-50 times on each side. (See picture, page 23, #5)

8. Patting the back: With a hollow palm, pat the opposite side of the upper back 30-50 times on each side. (See picture, page 23, #4 )

9. Nipping & kneading *He Gu* (LI 4): With the nail of
the opposite thumb, nip and knead *He Gu* (the
midpoint of the mound of muscle between
the thumb and index finger on the back of the
hand) approximately 100 times each side.

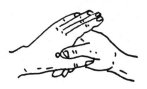

In addition, drink more hot water and get more rest. As soon as one feels one is catching a
cold, do the above self-massage 1-3 times a day. The results will be even better if this self-
massage is combined with Chinese herbal medicine.

## B. Headache

Headache refers to pain in the head. Although there are a number of different patterns of
headache in Chinese medicine, the basic statement about all pain is that, "If there is free flow,
there is no pain; if there is pain, there is no free flow." Therefore, Chinese self-massage for
headache emphasizes stimulating the main acupuncture points on the head and neck in
order to stimulate the circulation of the qi and blood. No matter why the qi and blood are
not flowing, if their flow is smoothed and eased, the pain will disappear.

**Massage methods:**

1. Pressing & kneading *Yin Tang* (M-HN-3):
With the thumb or middle finger of one hand,
press and knead *Yin Tang* (located at the
midpoint between the eyebrows)
approximately 100 times.

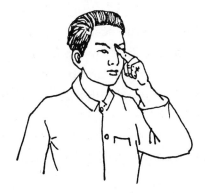

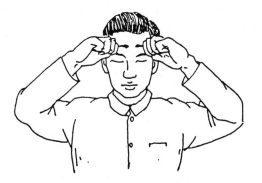

2. Pushing apart on the forehead: Bend the two index fingers and push with the lateral sides of their middle segments from the midline of the forehead between the eyebrows to the anterior hairline on both sides of the forehead, the corners of the forehead, and the ends of the eyebrows approximately 100 times.

3. Pressing & kneading *Tai Yang* (M-HN-9): With the tips of the thumbs or middle fingers, press and knead the paired points *Tai Yang* (located 1 body inch lateral to the lateral end of the eyebrow and the outer canthus) approximately 100 times until there is a sensation of mild soreness and distention.

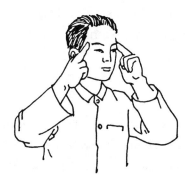

4. Wiping the temples: Place the pads of the thumbs on the corners of the forehead and wipe the temples backwards repeatedly with force approximately 100 times until there is a sensation of mild soreness and distention. (See picture, page 12, #2)

5. Grasping the top of the head: Place the tips of the five fingers of one hand on the forehead, the middle finger in the middle and the other four fingers at the sides. Grasp with them from the forehead to the top of the head 20-30 times.

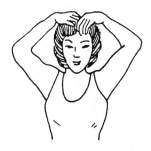

6. Patting the top of the head: Pat the top of the head with a hollow hand 30-50 times. (See picture, page 13, #4)

7. Pressing & kneading *Feng Chi* (GB 20): With the tips of both thumbs, press and knead the paired points *Feng Chi* (located in the depression between the sternocleidomastoid muscle

and the trapezius 1 body inch within the posterior hairline) approximately 100 times. (See picture, page 13, #3)

8. Grasping & pounding *Jian Jing* (GB 21): With the thumb, index, and middle fingers of each hand, grasp *Jian Jing* ( located at the midpoint on top of the shoulder) on the opposite side of the body 3-5 times each side. Then pound the point with an empty fist 30- 50 times each side.

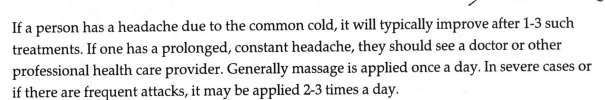

9. Pressing & kneading *Lie Que* (Lu 7): With the tip of the right thumb, press and knead the left *Lie Que* (located 1.5 cun above the transverse crease of the wrist on the radial side) approximately 100 times. Repeat this on the other side.

If a person has a headache due to the common cold, it will typically improve after 1-3 such treatments. If one has a prolonged, constant headache, they should see a doctor or other professional health care provider. Generally massage is applied once a day. In severe cases or if there are frequent attacks, it may be applied 2-3 times a day.

## C. Insomnia

In Chinese medicine, insomnia is basically due to an imbalance between yin and yang. It is the yang energy which opens the eyes and is responsible for consciousness. If yang is out of balance with yin and there is too much yang relative to yin, then one will not be able to go to sleep or will wake easily or early after going to sleep. Therefore, Chinese self-massage for insomnia mainly works by stimulating the production of yin and dispersing and leading yang qi downward. If insomnia is prolonged, other symptoms which may accompany it may include dizziness, headache, heart palpitations, forgetfulness, and restlessness. Since menopausal complaints are usually due to imbalance between yin and yang, insomnia often complicates perimenopausal syndrome.

**Massage methods:**

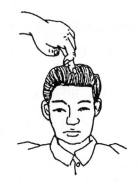

1. Pressing & kneading *Bai Hui* (GV 20): With the tip of the middle finger, press and knead *Bai Hui* (located in the middle of the top of the head at the midpoint on the line connecting the tips of both ears) approximately 100 times.

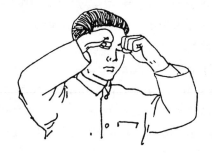

2. Kneading *Zan Zhu* (Bl 2): With the tips of the middle fingers, knead the paired points *Zan Zhu* (located in the depression just medial to the medial end of the eyebrow) 30-50 times.

3. Wiping the orbits: Bend the index fingers and wipe with the lateral sides of their middle segments on the upper and then lower orbits from the inner corners of the eyes to the outer 20-30 times.

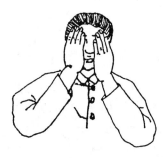

4. Heating the eyes: Close the eyes slightly. Rub the palms of the hands against each other until they become hot and then cover the eyes with the palms for 30-60 seconds, followed by lightly kneading them approximately 10 times.

5. Pressing & kneading *Feng Chi* (GB 20): With the tips of the thumbs, press and knead the paired points *Feng Chi* (located in the depression between the sternocleidomastoid muscle and the trapezius 1 body inch within the posterior hairline) 30-50 times. ( See picture, page 13, #3)

6. Circular rubbing *Zhong Wan* (CV 12) and *Guan Yuan* (CV 4): With one palm, circularly rub *Zhong Wan* (located at the midpoint of the upper abdomen) and *Guan Yuan* (located at the midpoint of the lower abdomen) clockwise approximately 100 times and then counterclockwise 100 times for each point. (See picture, page 60, #2)

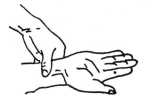

7. Pressing & kneading *Nei Guan* (Per 6): With the right thumb, press and knead the left *Nei Guan* (located 2 body inches above the midpoint of the transverse crease of the wrist on the palmar surface of the forearm) 30-50 times. Repeat this on the opposite side.

8. Pressing & kneading *Shen Men* (Ht 7): With the tip of the right thumb, press and knead the left *Shen Men* (located on the ulnar side of the transverse crease of the wrist on the palm surface) 30-50 times. Repeat this on the opposite side.

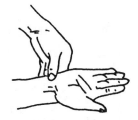

9. Pressing & kneading *Zu San Li* (St 36): Press and knead with the thumb on the point 3 body inches below the outside lower edge of the kneecap 30-50 times on each leg. (See picture, page 60, #4)

10. Pressing & kneading *San Yin Jiao* (Sp 6): Press and knead the point 3 body inches above the tip of the inner ankle on the posterior border of the medial aspect of the tibia 30-50 times on each leg.

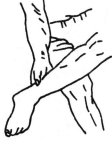

11. Rubbing *Yong Quan* (Ki 1): With the fleshy pad of muscle at the base of the little finger, rub rapidly and forcefully on the sole of the opposite foot at the point *Yong Quan* (located in the depression lateral to the ball of the foot) until there is a hot feeling. Repeat this on the other foot. (See picture, page 60, #5)

When going to bed, one should quietly lie on the bed, relaxing all over the body and getting rid of distracting thoughts. One should not drink strong tea or coffee after midday but can try drinking some warm milk before going to bed. Pay attention to getting regular exercise, building up health and improving physical and mental health. It is best to do this self-massage in the evening before going to bed. Quietly rest 15-30 minutes after the self-massage. Then go to bed and naturally fall asleep. If one has not slept during the night, one should not sleep in late or nap during the day trying to make up for the lost sleep. This will only throw one's sleep-wake cycle further off.

## D. Dizziness

In Chinese medicine, dizziness may be due to three basic mechanisms. First, yang may come out of balance with yin and counterflow or rebel frenetically upward causing a kind of internal wind in the head. Secondly, there may be insufficient yang qi and/or yin blood to nourish and empower the brain. This is especially the case if dizziness occurs when one stands up quickly. One feels as if they are going to black out because the qi and blood have not risen with the body to empower the brain's function. The third reason for dizziness is too much phlegm in the body. This phlegm may block the orifices or portals of the head, thus preventing the qi and blood from nourishing and empowering the brain. The Chinese self-massage mechanisms described below primarily work by quickening the blood and moving the qi in the region of the head, thus sweeping away obstruction and allowing upwardly counterflowing qi to find its way out of the head.

Dizziness may often be seen in Meniere's syndrome, cerebral arteriosclerosis, hypertension, anemia, and some brain diseases. Therefore, if this self-massage regime does not help the dizziness in a timely and adequate way, one should see a professional health care practitioner for a more complete and accurate diagnosis and treatment. Both acupuncture and Chinese herbal medicine treat most kinds of dizziness quite effectively.

**Massage methods:**

1. Opening heaven's gate: Push upward along the midline of the forehead with the index and middle fingers of both hands alternately beginning at the midpoint between the eyebrows up to the anterior hairline 50-100 times. Push in one direction only, *i.e.*, upward.

2. Pushing apart on the forehead: Bend the two index fingers and push with the lateral sides of their middle segments from the midline of the forehead which runs from the midpoint between the eyebrows to the anterior hairline on both sides of the forehead and the ends of the eyebrows altogether approximately 100 times.

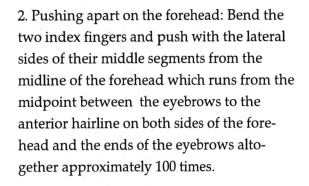

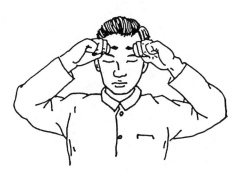

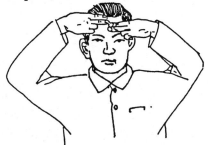

3. Kneading *Tai Yang* (M-HN-9): Press with the tip of the thumbs or middle fingers on the points *Tai Yang* (located 1 body inch lateral to the lateral end of each eyebrow and outer canthus and then knead them approximately 100 times until there is a sensation of mild soreness and distention.

4. Sweeping the temples: With the tips of the five fingers held close together, rub the right temple from the corner of the forehead to the bulging bone behind the ear 30-50 times. Then rub the left temple an equal number of times.

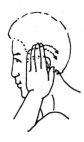

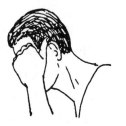

5. Pressing & kneading *Jiao Sun* (TB 20): With the tips of both thumbs, separately press and knead the points above the tips of the ears at the hairline 30-50 times.

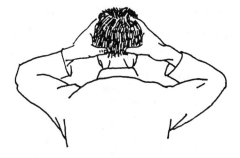

6. Pressing & kneading *Feng Chi* (GB 20): With the tips of both thumbs, press and knead the paired points *Feng Chi* (located in the depression between the sternocleidomastoid muscle and the trapezius 1 body inch superior to the posterior hairline) 30-50 times.

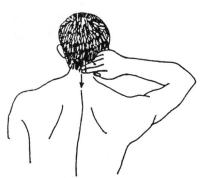

7. Pushing the heavenly pillar bones: With the index and middle fingers of one hand held close together, push in one direction only from the posterior hairline to the bulging bone at the base of the neck approximately 100 times.

When there is dizziness, it is important to try to keep the mind relaxed, avoiding mental irritation as much as possible. Establish a proper balance between work and rest and be moderate in sexual intercourse. Avoid eating and drinking too much at one meal and eating too much fatty and/or sweet foods. One should also give up smoking and stop drinking alcohol. The above Chinese self-massage routine should be done once per day. Then rest for several minutes after the completion of these manipulations. This self-massage may be done before going to bed at night.

# E. Hypertension

Hypertension means high blood pressure. It is a common chronic disease mainly characterized by the continuous increase of arterial pressure. It is also called essential hypertension. Hypertension is usually defined as blood pressure higher than 140/90 in those under 40 years of age, more than 150/90 in those 40-59, and more than 160/90 in those over 60 years old. The degree of symptoms of hypertension varies greatly. Some patients may have no subjective symptoms. The only way they know their blood pressure is high is by taking it with a blood pressure cuff. However, many people with hypertension experience the symptoms of dizziness, headache, flushing, conjunctival congestion, a bitter taste in the mouth, heart palpitations, and constipation. Some patients may also have the symptoms of tinnitus, vexation, forgetfulness, lassitude in loins and legs, nausea, poor appetite, an oppressed or tight, stuffy feeling in the chest, insomnia, and dream-disturbed sleep. This disease has a high incidence and is often related to age, profession, and family history. Chinese self- massage is very effective for stabilizing blood pressure as long as high blood pressure is not due to organic disease. Like dizziness, high blood pressure is mostly due to a yin/yang imbalance, with yang being hyperactive and flushing or counterflowing upward in the body. Therefore, Chinese self-massage manipulations for hypertension mostly are aimed at subduing yang, supplementing yin, and reversing counterflow.

**Massage methods:**

1. Pressing & kneading *Yin Tang* (M-HN-3):
With the thumb or middle finger of one hand,
press and knead *Yin Tang* (located at the
midpoint between the eyebrows)
30-50 times.

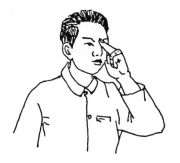

2. Pressing & kneading *Tai Yang* (M-HN-9): Press with the tip of the thumbs or middle fingers on the points *Tai Yang* (located 1 body inch lateral to the lateral end of each eyebrow

and outer canthus) and knead them 30-50 times until there is a sensation of mild soreness and distention. (See picture, page 75, #3)

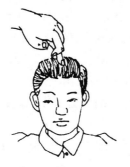

3. Pressing & kneading *Bai Hui* (GV 20): With the tip of the middle finger, press and knead *Bai Hui* (located at the middle of the top of the head at the midpoint on the line connecting the tips of both ears) 30-50 times.

4. Pressing & kneading *Feng Chi* (GB 20): With the tips of the thumbs, press and knead the paired points *Feng Chi* (located in the depression between the sternocleidomastoid muscle and trapezius 1 body inch superior to the posterior hairline) 30-50 times. (See picture, page 76, #6)

5. Pushing *Qiao Gong*: With the thumb, push the line on the neck on the same side of the body from the bulging bone behind the ear to the center of the supraclavicular fossa 30-50 times. Then push the other side of the neck with the other thumb the same number of times.

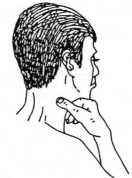

6. Circular rubbing the navel: With one palm, circularly rub the navel and abdomen around the navel clockwise for approximately 5 minutes. (See picture, page 37, #4)

7. Rubbing the lateral costal region: With both palms, rub the lateral costal region from the armpits to the sides of the navel to produce a sensation of heat.

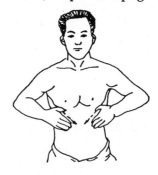

8. Pounding *Jian Jing* (GB 21): With a hollow fist, pound the point at the midpoint of the top of the shoulder on the opposite side of the body alternately 30-50 times on each side.

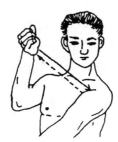

9. Patting the back: With hollow palms, pat the opposite side of the upper back alternately 30-50 times on each side. (See picture, page 23, #4)

10. Pressing & kneading *Qu Chi* (LI 11) and *Nei Guan* (Per 6): With the tip of the right thumb, press and knead the left *Qu Chi* (located at the lateral end of the transverse elbow crease when the elbow is flexed) and then the left *Nei Guan* (located 2 body inches above the midpoint of the transverse wrist crease on the palmar surface of the forearm) 30- 50 times. Repeat these maneuvers on the points on the right arm.

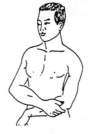
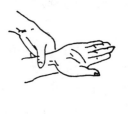

11. Pressing & kneading *Zu San Li* (St 36) and *San Yin Jiao* (Sp 6): With the tips of both thumbs, press and knead *Zu San Li* (located 3 body inches below the lateral side of the lower, outer edge of the kneecap) and *San Yin Jiao* (located 3 body inches above the tip of the inner ankle) 30-50 times on each point on each leg. (See picture, page 60, #4)

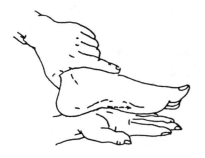

12. Rubbing *Yong Quan* (Ki 1): With the fleshy pad of muscle at the base of the little finger, rub rapidly and forcefully on the sole of the opposite foot the point *Yong Quan* (located in the depression lateral to the ball of the foot) producing a hot feeling.

For those with hypertension, it is very important to get regular exercise. It is also important not to allow oneself to get over-fatigued. As much as possible, avoid mental irritation, and do not eat any greasy, fatty foods or drink alcohol. The above self-massage regimen should be done once per day.

## F. Coronary heart disease

Coronary heart disease, also called coronary atherosclerotic cardiopathy, is one of the common diseases of the middle-aged and elderly. In its early or remission stages, there may not be any symptoms. However, during physical examination, the patient may be found to have high cholesterol and an EKG may show myocardial ischemia. These indicate that coronary atherosclerosis exists and this is called latent coronary heart disease.

A typical patient may manifest paroxysmal pain in the area behind the sternum and in front of the heart. This pain may refer to the shoulder, arm, and upper back and is then called angina pectoris. The symptoms of heart palpitations, chest oppression, and shortness of breath may accompany this pain and a feeling of asphyxiation may present in severe cases. These symptoms may last several minutes before they disappear. In severe cases, life may be in danger during such an attack. At other times, the patient may have the symptoms of dizziness, tinnitus, low back soreness, listlessness, poor appetite, dull facial complexion, etc.

Although persons with coronary heart disease should be under the care of professional health care practitioners, Chinese self-massage can dilate the blood vessels, reduce the obstruction of arterial blood flow, thus relieving the heart's stress and improving the blood supply to the coronary arteries. Thus such Chinese self-massage can effectively help prevent and treat coronary heart disease.

Although there are a number of different patterns of coronary heart disease in Chinese medicine, each requiring their own special treatments with acupuncture or Chinese herbal medicine, the Chinese self-massage maneuvers below primarily work to open the flow of qi and blood in the chest and to supplement and regulate the heart, liver, stomach, and intestines.

**Massage methods:**

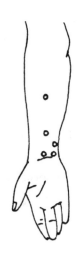

1. Pressing & kneading the points on the upper limbs: With the tip of each thumb, press and knead the points *Da Ling* (Per 7, located at the midpoint of the transverse wrist crease on the palmar surface of the wrist), *Shen Men* (Ht 7, located on the ulnar side of the transverse wrist crease on the palmar surface of the wrist), *Tong Li* (Ht 5, located 1 body inch above *Shen Men*), *Nei Guan* (Per 6, located 2 body inches above *Da Ling*), and *Xi Men* (Per 4, located 5 body inches above *Da Ling*) on the opposite arm approximately 100 times each point.

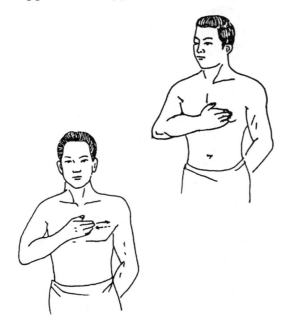

2. Kneading & circular rubbing the precordium: Place the center of the palm of the right hand lightly on the precordium (the area of the left nipple). Then knead and circularly rub the area clockwise 3-5 times.

3. Rubbing the chest: With one palm, transversely rub the chest to and fro to produce a hot sensation.

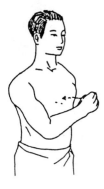

4. Patting the chest: With the hollow of the palm, lightly pat both sides of the chest approximately 100 times.

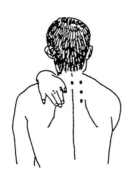

5. Pressing & kneading *Xin Shu* (Bl 15) and *Jue Yin Shu* (Bl 14): With the tips of both middle fingers, press and knead the paired points *Xin Shu* (located 1.5 body inches lateral to the lower edge of the 5th thoracic vertebra) and *Jue Yin Shu* (located 1.5 body inches lateral to the lower edge of the 4th thoracic vertebra) approximately 100 times each point.

6. Pounding the back: With the back of a hollow fist, pound the back 100-200 times.

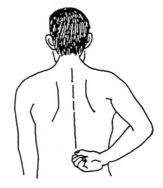

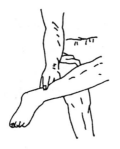

7. Pressing & kneading *Zu San Li* (St 36) and *San Yin Jiao* (Sp 6): With the tips of both thumbs, press and knead *Zu San Li* (located 3 body inches below the lower, outer edge of the kneecap) and *San Yin Jiao* (located 3 body inches above the tip of the inner ankle) 30-50 times each point on each leg.

People suffering from coronary heart disease should try to keep their peace of mind and cultivate a stable mood. They should avoid catching cold, and should eat what is called in Chinese medicine a clear, bland diet. They should avoid, greasy, fatty foods and sugars and sweets. They should try to strike a proper balance between work and rest and get regular physical exercise. The amount of this exercise should be increased gradually. However, exercise should not be increased during periods of frequent angina pectoris attacks. The main exercise should be walking. In addition, daily deep relaxation exercises should be practiced in either the sitting or lying position.

At the time of an angina pectoris attack, one should first press and knead *Nei Guan* and *Xi Men* on both arms 100-200 times for each point or until the attack is relieved. This can be done in conjunction with taking nitroglycerine tablets or other prescribed heart medication. Acupuncture and Chinese herbal medicine are both effective for treating coronary heart disease which may be used as adjuncts to modern Western medicine.

## G. Cough

Cough is one of the main symptoms of respiratory system disease. Many diseases such as the common cold, bronchitis, pneumonia, pulmonary emphysema, and pulmonary tuberculosis can cause coughing. Here in this book, cough refers to acute and chronic bronchitis whose main symptom is cough. Chinese self-massage can relieve this symptom, enhance the body's immunity, and speed the body's recovery. In Chinese medicine there are close to a dozen different patterns associated with cough. However, cough itself is seen as an upward counterflow of the lung qi and a loss of the lungs' spreading and diffusing function. Therefore, the Chinese self-massage maneuvers given below mainly reverse lung counterflow and loosen and spread the lung qi.

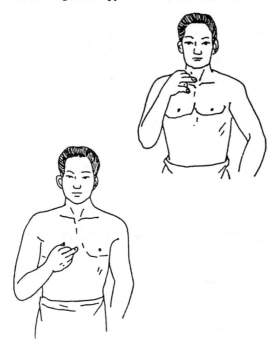

**Massage methods:**

1. Pressing & kneading *Tian Tu* (CV 22): With the tip of the middle finger, press and knead the point at the center of the suprasternal fossa approximately 100 times.

2. Pressing & kneading *Shan Zhong* (CV 17): With the tip of the middle finger, press and knead *Shan Zhong* (located on the chest between the two nipples in males) 100-200 times.

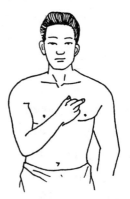

3. Pressing & kneading *Zhong Fu* (Lu 1): With the tips of both middle fingers, press and knead *Zhong Fu* (located 6 body inches lateral to the midline of the chest in the interspace between the 1st and 2nd ribs on both sides of the chest) 100-200 times each point.

4. Rubbing the chest: With one palm, rub the chest to and fro transversely until there is a feeling of heat.

5. Pressing & kneading *Feng Men* (Bl 12) and *Fei Shu* (Bl 13): With the tips of both middle fingers, press and knead the points 1.5 body inches lateral to the lower edges of the 2nd and 3rd thoracic vertebrae approximately 100 times each point.

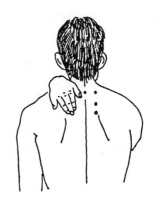

Persons with cough should keep themselves warm and avoid catching cold. Do not eat any spicy, greasy food or dairy products such as milk and cheese and do not smoke or drink alcohol. Although acupuncture can help relieve cough, Chinese herbal medicine is particularly effective for treating cough and upper respiratory diseases in general. The reader can see *The Book of Jook: Chinese Medicinal Porridges; Chinese Medicinal Wines & Elixirs;* or *Chinese Medicinal Teas,* all published by Blue Poppy Press, for simple Chinese home remedies and herbal formulas for treating cough due to the common cold and bronchitis.

## H. Asthma

Asthma refers to shortness of breath, wheezing, breathing with an open mouth and raised shoulders, and difficulty lying on one's back in severe cases. Asthma can be either a disease in its own right — bronchial or allergic asthma — or it can be a symptom of various heart and lung diseases. The Chinese self-massage maneuvers given in this book are meant for bronchial or allergic asthma.

Bronchial asthma is a common disease characterized by sudden, repeated episodes of wheezing, shortness of breath, and difficulty breathing. These attacks are typically provoked by certain allergens, exercise, or climatic changes. Before the onset of such an attack, some patients experience the prodromal symptoms of sneezing, itching in the nose and the throat, and discomfort in the chest. However, an asthma attack can also occur suddenly without such premonitory signs and symptoms. The major symptoms of this disease are stuffiness in the chest and rapid breathing with wheezing. Patient's with this disease typically have to sit up during an attack. In severe cases, there are the symptoms of flaring of the nostrils when trying to breathe, breathing with an open mouth, and raising the shoulders when breathing. There may also be cyanotic lips and nails due to lack of oxygen. When the attack is relieved, the patient will initially cough up some frothy mucoid sputum. This disease can occur repeatedly with the complications of pulmonary emphysema and pulmonary heart disease.

During the remission stage, persons with asthma usually have such symptoms as intolerance to cold, spontaneous perspiration, abundant expectoration of phlegm, poor appetite, shortness of breath, lassitude in the loins and legs, a feverish sensation in the palms of the hands and soles of the feet, and night sweats.

Although there are a number of different patterns of asthma in Chinese medicine, asthma is mainly seen as a lung, spleen, and kidney disease complicated by excessive phlegm. Because of a breakdown in the interaction between the lungs and kidneys, the lung qi counterflows upward and does not spread and descend downward as it should. In addition, because of poor spleen function, the body produces too much phlegm and dampness which accumulates in the lungs and also impedes the lungs clearing and diffusing function. Thus respiration becomes blocked and obstructed. Based on this vision of this disease's mechanisms, the Chinese self-massage manipulations below are mainly aimed at spreading and descending the lung qi, transforming and eliminating dampness, and supplementing or strengthening the spleen and kidneys.

**Massage methods:**

1. Pressing & kneading *Tian Tu* (CV 22): With the tip of the middle finger, press and knead the point at the center of the notch above the sternum or breast bone approximately 100 times.

2. Pressing & kneading *Shan Zhong* (CV 17): With the tip of the middle finger, press and knead *Shan Zhong* (located in the middle of the chest between the two nipples in males) 100-200 times.

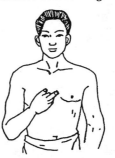

3. Pressing & kneading *Ding Chuan* (M-BW-1b) and *Fei Shu* (Bl 13): With the tips of both middle fingers, press and knead *Ding Chuan* (located 0.5 body inch lateral to the bulging bone at the base of the neck) and *Fei Shu* (located 1.5 body inches lateral to the 3rd thoracic vertebra) approximately 100 times each point.

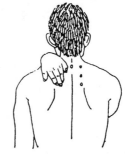

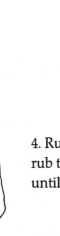

4. Rubbing the chest: With one palm, rub the chest to and fro transversely until there is a feeling of heat.

5. Circular rubbing the abdomen: With one palm, circularly rub the abdomen around the navel for approximately 3-5 minutes.

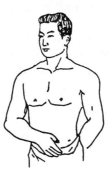

6. Pressing & kneading *Qi Hai* (CV 6) and *Guan Yuan* (CV 4): With the heel of one palm, press and knead the points 1.5 body inches and 3 body inches below the navel 100-200 times each point.

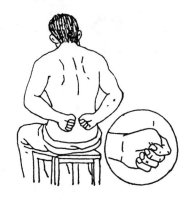

7. Pressing & kneading *Pi Shu* (Bl 20) and *Shen Shu* (Bl 23): With the bent knuckles of both thumbs, press and knead *Pi Shu* (located 1.5 body inches lateral to the lower edge of the 11th thoracic vertebra) and *Shen Shu* (located 1.5 body inches lateral to the lower edge of the 2nd lumbar vertebra) 100-200 times each point.

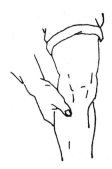

8. Pressing & kneading *Zu San Li* (St 36) and *Feng Long* (St 40): With the tips of both thumbs, press and knead *Zu San Li* (located 3 body inches below the lower, outside edge of the kneecap) and *Feng Long* (located 8 body inches above the tip of the outside ankle at the midpoint between the lateral side of the knee and the ankle) 30- 50 times each point.

During an asthmatic attack, first press and knead *Tian Tu, Shan Zhong, Ding Chuan,* and *Fei Shu* with strong force. Massage the other points during the remission stage to help prevent recurrent attacks. During the remission stage, if one combines self-massage with moxibustion on *Qi Hai* (CV 6), *Guan Yuan* (CV 4), *Da Zhui* (GV 14), *Fei Shu* (Bl 13), *Pi Shu* (Bl 20), and *Shen Shu* (Bl 23) for 3-5 minutes each point, the effect will be much better. One can learn how to do moxibustion on these points from a local, professional acupuncturist.

Otherwise, keep warm and avoid catching cold to prevent an attack which may be induced by catching cold. Eat a hypoallergenic, yeast-free, clear, bland diet. Do not eat any food which is greasy, pungent, overly salty, or overly sweet. Do not eat fish and shrimp, and do not drink alcohol. For more information on such a yeast-free, hypoallergenic, clear, bland diet, see Bob Flaws's *Arisal of the Clear: A Simple Guide to Healthy Eating According to Traditional*

*Chinese Medicine.* Unless asthma is induced by exercise, do more physical exercise to build up one's health, give up smoking, and moderate your sexual life.

## I. Hiccup

Hiccup refers to the uncontrollable persistent repetition of sharp, gulp-like sounds from the throat. They are caused by repeated involuntary contraction of the diaphragm due to stimulation of the vagus and phrenic nerves. The major causes of hiccups are nervous excitement, quick and  excessive eating, and sudden breathing in of cold air. Hiccups may also occur in diseases such as stomach cancer and hysteria, during pregnancy, or after surgical operation. In most cases, however, hiccups are purely functional and can be quickly cured by Chinese self-massage. In Chinese medicine, just as cough is seen as an upward counterflow of the lung qi, hiccups are due to upward counterflow of stomach qi. Therefore, the following Chinese self-massage maneuvers for hiccup are mainly aimed at reversing the direction of the flow of the stomach qi.

**Massage methods:**

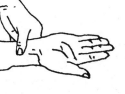

1. Pressing & kneading *Nei Guan* (Per 6) and *He Gu* (LI 4): With the tip of the right thumb, press and knead the left *Nei Guan* (located 2 body inches above the midpoint of the transverse wrist crease on the palmar surface of the forearm) and *He Gu* (located at the midpoint of the bulge in the angle between the thumb and index finger) 100-200 times each. Then repeat these maneuvers on the left side.

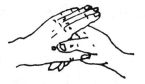

2. Pressing & kneading *Zan Zhu* (Bl 2) and *Shuai Gu* (GB 8): Place the tips of both thumbs on *Zan Zhu* (located in the depression medial to the medial end of the eyebrow) on both sides

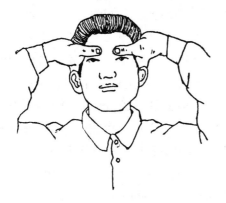

and put the other closed four fingers of both hands on *Shuai Gu* (located above the apex of the ear and 1.5 body inches above the hairline) on both sides of the head. First press and knead and then press with strong force until there is an obvious feeling of soreness and distention around these points. Keep pressing like this for approximately 5 minutes.

3. Pressing and kneading *Shan Zhong* (CV 17): With the tip of the middle finger, press and knead *Shan Zhong* (located at the midpoint of the chest between the two nipples in males) 100-200 times.

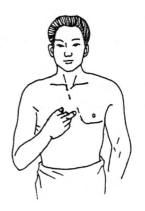

4. Patting the chest: With one hollow palm, lightly pat both sides of the chest and both sides of the costal regions 100-200 times. (See picture, page 82, #4)

5. Holding the breath: Breathe in deeply and hold the breath as long as possible before breathing out. Generally, hiccups can be stopped after holding the breath like this for 3-5 times.

## J. Vomiting

Vomiting is a common clinical symptom which may be caused by many factors. It can be seen in many diseases, such as gastritis, neurogenic vomiting, spasm of the pylorus, pylorochesis, cholecystitis, and urinary tract stones. Light vomiting or constant vomiting due to prolonged diseases can be relieved quickly with Chinese self-massage in most cases. If vomiting is accompanied by abdominal pain, high fever, and unclear mind due to poisoning or acute abdominal conditions, such as appendicitis or urinary tract stones, the patient should see their Western MD or go to a hospital emergency room as soon as possible.

In Chinese medicine, vomiting is very much like hiccup in that both are the manifestation of upwardly counterflowing stomach qi. Therefore, the Chinese self-massage manipulations described below all mainly reverse and descend the stomach counterflow.

**Massage methods:**

1. Pressing & kneading *Qu Chi* (LI 11) and *Nei Guan* (Per 6): With the tip of the thumb of the right hand, press and knead the left *Qu Chi* (located at the lateral end of the transverse elbow crease when the elbow is flexed) and *Nei Guan* (located 2 body inches above the midpoint of the transverse wrist crease on the palmar surface of the forearm) approximately 100 times each. Then repeat this process on the right side.

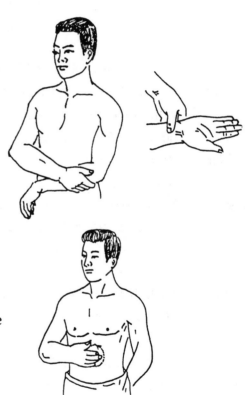

2. Circular rubbing *Zhong Wan* (CV 12): With one palm, circularly rub *Zhong Wan* (located 4 body inches above the navel, midway between the navel and the lower tip of the sternum) clockwise for approximately 5 minutes.

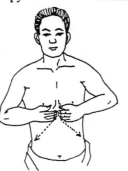

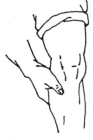

3. Pushing apart *Zhong* Wan: Place the four fingers of both hands on the two sides of the midpoint of the upper abdomen. The four fingers should be held closely together. Then push apart obliquely to the sides of the abdomen 100-200 times.

4. Pressing & kneading *Zu San Li* (St 36): With the tips of both thumbs, press and knead *Zu San Li* (located 3 body inches below the lower, outside edge of the kneecap) approximately 100 times each.

5. Pressing & kneading *Pi Shu* (Bl 20) and *Wei Shu* (Bl 22): With the bent knuckles of both thumbs, press and knead *Pi Shu* (located 1.5 body inches lateral to the lower edge of the 11th thoracic vertebra) and *Wei Shu* (located 1.5 body inches lateral to the lower edge of the 12th thoracic vertebra) 100-200 times each.

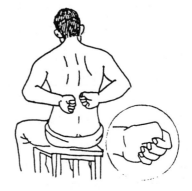

Persons with vomiting, including women with morning sickness, should eat several small meals rather than only a couple of large meals per day. In addition, the meals should consist of light, easily digestible foods. If vomiting persists, one should definitely see a professional health care practitioner. Acupuncture and Chinese herbal medicine both treat vomiting quite well, including morning sickness.

## K. Stomachache

Stomachache mainly manifests as frequent pain in the upper abdomen. It may be caused by over-eating raw and cold food, catching cold, emotional anguish, or over-fatigue. It can be seen in many digestive tract diseases, such as gastritis, stomach or duodenal ulcers, gastroptosis, gastroneurosis, stomach spasm, etc. Chinese self-massage can relieve stomachache as well as improve the function of digestion. It can also treat certain organic diseases such as stomach and duodenal ulcers. However, self-massage should not be used during episodes of bleeding due to stomach or duodenal ulcers, in which case, the main symptoms are black, tarry stools, vomiting blood, and hematochezia. In Chinese medicine, since all pain is seen as a manifestation of a lack of free flow of the qi and blood, the Chinese self-massage maneuvers given below mainly quicken the blood and move the qi in the epigastrium and regulate the functions of the viscera and bowels associated with digestion.

**Massage methods:**

1. Circular rubbing *Zhong Wan* (CV 12): With one palm, circularly rub the midpoint of the upper abdomen 100-200 times. (See picture, page 91, #2 )

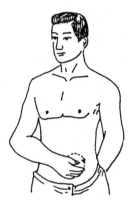

2. Circular rubbing the abdomen: With one palm, circularly rub the abdomen around the navel ➡ 100-200 times.

3. Pushing apart the abdomen: With the pads of the four fingers of both hands, push apart the abdomen beginning from the angle below the sternum, then the midpoint of the upper abdomen, and then the navel to the sides of the abdomen 30-50 times altogether.

4. Pressing & kneading *Zhong Wan* (CV 12), *Liang Men* (St 21), and *Tian Shu* (St 25): With the tip of the middle finger of one hand, press and knead *Zhong Wan* (located at the midpoint of the upper abdomen). Then, with the tips of the middle fingers of both hands, press and knead *Liang Men* (located 2 body inches lateral to *Zhong Wan*) and *Tian Shu* (located 2 body inches lateral to the navel) 30-50 times each.

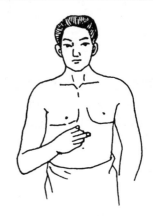

5. Pressing & kneading *Pi Shu* (Bl 20) and *Wei Shu* (Bl 22): With the bent knuckles of both thumbs, press and knead *Pi Shu* (located 1.5 body inches lateral to the lower edge of the 11th thoracic vertebra) and *Wei Shu* (located 1. 5 body inches lateral to the lower edge of the 12th thoracic vertebra) 100-200 times each. (See picture, page 88, #7)

6. Pressing & kneading *Zu San Li* (St 36): With the tips of both thumbs, press and knead *Zu San Li* (located 3 body inches below the lower, outside edge of the kneecap) approximately 100 times each. (See picture, page 88, # 8)

If there is a severe stomachache, you should first find by feeling around and press the tender point which is near *Pi Shu* or *Wei Shu* on the back with strong force for approximately 2 minutes. After the pain is relieved, you can then massage yourself according to the above procedures. One should regulate their life, being moderate in eating and drinking. Do not eat any food which is raw, cold, or spicy. Rather, one should eat food which is light and easy to digest or may eat more meals per day but less food at each meal. Keep a happy mood and do not get over-fatigued. If Chinese self-massage does not relieve the stomachache either adequately or in a timely manner or if stomachache continues to recur even after changing one's diet and lifestyle, one should see a professional health care practitioner.

## L. Diarrhea

Diarrhea refers to an increase in the frequency of bowel movements per day, loose stools, and even watery stools. There are many causes of diarrhea, such as germs, improper diet, mental-emotional factors, and weakness of the functions of the digestive system. Diarrhea can also be divided into acute and chronic types. Acute diarrhea occurs as a sudden attack, is severe with very frequent bowel movements possibly containing mucus, and is commonly accompanied by nausea, vomiting, abdominal pain, fever, etc. In most cases, it is caused by germs and so-called food poisoning. Chronic diarrhea may either develop from prolonged acute diarrhea or may occur due to emotional causes, improper diet, or chronic imbalance of the intestinal flora and fauna. It has a long course and is accompanied by symptoms of general weakness and/or mental-emotional symptoms.

The Chinese self-massage maneuvers described below are most effective for chronic diarrhea. For acute diarrhea or for chronic diarrhea which does not respond to this self-massage regimen, Chinese herbal medicine is usually very effective. The self-massage maneuvers below seek to supplement and regulate the spleen, stomach, large intestine, and the kidneys, the main viscera and bowels associated with chronic diarrhea in Chinese medicine.

**Massage methods:**

1. Circular rubbing the points on the abdomen: With one palm, circularly rub around *Zhong Wan* (CV 12, located at the midpoint of the upper abdomen), *Shen Que* (CV 8, the navel), *Qi Hai* (CV 6, located 1.5 body inches below the navel), and *Guan Yuan* (CV 4, located 3 body inches below the navel) counterclockwise for approximately 3-5 minutes each.

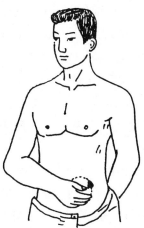

2. Pressing & kneading the points on the back: With the bent knuckles of both thumbs, press and knead the points *Pi Shu* (Bl 20, located 1.5 body inches lateral to the lower edge of the 11th thoracic vertebra), *Wei Shu* (Bl 21, located 1.5 body inches lateral to the lower edge of the 12th thoracic vertebra), *Shen Shu* (Bl 23, located 1.5 body inches lateral to the lower edge of the 2nd lumbar vertebra), and *Da Chang Shu* (Bl 25, located 1.5 body inches lateral to the lower edge of the 4th lumbar vertebra) approximately 100 times each. (See picture page 92, #5)

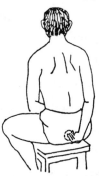

3. Pressing & kneading *Chang Qiang* (GV 1): With the tip of the middle finger of one hand, press and knead *Chang Qiang* (located 0.5 body inches below the tip of the tailbone) approximately 100 times.

4. Pressing & kneading *Zu San Li* (St 36): With the tips of both thumbs, press and knead *Zu San Li* (located 3 body inches below the lower, outside edge of the kneecap) approximately 100 times each. (See picture, page 88, #5)

Persons with diarrhea should not eat any food containing much fat. Also, do not eat any food which is raw, cold, chilled, and hard to digest. In Chinese medicine, the process of digestion is likened to the process of cooking, but on the inside of the body. Before digestion can be commenced, all food must be turned into 100°F soup within the stomach. Many Westerners suffer from chronic loose stools or undigested food within their stools and the chronic fatigue and bodily heaviness which goes along with these due to over-eating raw foods, such as salads, and chilled, cold foods and drinks out of the refrigerator, such as iced water and tea, frozen yogurt, and ice cream. These chilled, raw foods damage the spleen and stomach and ultimately injure the kidneys as well. Bob Flaws, in his *Arisal of the Clear: A Simple Guide to Healthy Eating According to Traditional Chinese Medicine*, discusses at length the importance of eating cooked, warm food.

Some middle-aged and elderly people with chronic diarrhea usually have loose stools before dawn each day. In Chinese medicine, this is called fifth watch or cockcrow diarrhea. People with diarrhea before dawn should eat only a very little and only easily digested food for supper. For this type of diarrhea associated with kidney weakness in Chinese medicine, moxibustion at *Shen Shu* (Bl 23) and *Ming Men* (GV 4) can make Chinese self-massage even more effective. This can be learned from a local professional acupuncturist.

## M. Constipation

Constipation refers to difficulty defecating, prolongation of time between bowel movements, and small, hard, desiccated stools. Some people may go 3-5 days or longer between bowel movements. Constipation is mainly caused by the abnormal conduction of the large intestine, too long of feces within the intestine, and too much moisture being reabsorbed by the large intestine thus resulting in dry, solid stools. Constipation can be found in various diseases and may also be due to lack of exercise, irregular lifestyle, lack of roughage in the diet, and irregular bowel movements which weaken intestinal peristalsis and thus causing constipation. Chinese self-massage can strengthen gastrointestinal peristalsis, regulate gastrointestinal function, and strengthen the powers of abdominal muscles so as to treat constipation with very good effects. According to Chinese medical theory, the self-massage manipulations described below mainly regulate and strengthen the functions of the spleen, stomach, large intestine, and kidneys, and lead the qi to move downward, thus opening the bowels.

**Massage methods:**

1. Circular rubbing the abdomen: With one palm, circularly rub the abdomen around the navel clockwise for 5-10 minutes. (See picture, page 93, #2)

2. Pressing & kneading *Tian Shu* (St 25): With the tips of the middle fingers of both hands, press and knead *Tian Shu* (located 2 body inches lateral to the navel) 100-200 times. ➡

3. Pressing & kneading the points on the back: With the bent knuckles of both thumbs, press and knead the points *Pi Shu* (Bl 20, located 1.5 body inches lateral to the lower edge of the 11th thoracic vertebra), *Wei Shu* (Bl 21, located 1.5 body inches lateral to the lower edge of the 12th thoracic vertebra), *Shen Shu* (Bl 23, located 1.5 body inches lateral to the lower edge of the 2nd lumbar vertebra), and *Da Chang Shu* (Bl 25, located 1.5 body inches lateral to the lower edge of the 4th lumbar vertebra) approximately 100 times each. (See picture, page 92, #5)

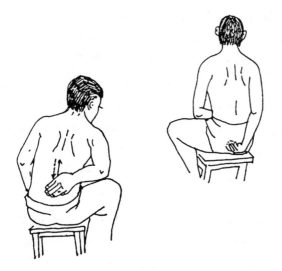

4. Pressing & kneading *Chang Qiang* (GV 1): With the tip of the middle finger of one hand, press and knead *Chang Qiang* (located 0.5 body inches below the tip of the tailbone) 100-200 times

5. Rubbing the lumbosacral area: Place one palm on the middle of the low back. Rub the midline of the lower part of the spine up and down 30-50 times to produce a sensation of heat.

6. Pressing & kneading *Zhi Gou* (TB 6): With the tip of the right thumb, press and knead the left *Zhi Gou* (located 3 body inches above the midpoint of the transverse crease of the wrist on the back of the forearm) approximately 100 times. Then repeat on the other side.

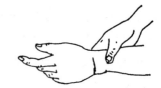

Persons with habitual constipation should pay attention to regulating their diet. One should eat more vegetables, fruits, and foods which are high in roughage. Do not eat any foods which are spicy and irritating. Also one should drink more water. In addition, one should try to form a regular habit of having a bowel movement each morning. One should not abuse purgatives as these may damage the large intestine and become addictive. Adequate physical exercise is important to keep the abdominal muscles strong and for insuring the smooth and free flow of qi. Since sluggish large intestine function and its consequent constipation are associated with the onset of many diseases, keeping the bowels open and freely moving with Chinese self-massage is one simple, free, yet very effective way of preventing many common chronic diseases.

## N. Cholecystitis & cholelithiasis

Cholecystitis or gallbladder colic is a digestive tract disease. It often occurs in middle-aged women who are overweight. Its main manifest is a paroxysmal pain in the right upper abdomen which may gradually change into a continuous pain with paroxysmal exacerbations. This pain may radiate to the right upper back. The main reason for this pain is biliary tract obstruction and blocked excretion of bile. This blockage of the bile ducts is mainly due to the presence of gallstones. Modern research has shown that gallstones are present in virtually all cases of gallbladder inflammation and colic.

Cholecystitis is divided into acute and chronic types. Acute cholecystitis often attacks after a large meal or after eating greasy food. These attacks are also more common in the evening or at midnight when Chinese medicine says the gallbladder is at high tide. Besides pain in the right upper abdomen possibly radiating to the right scapula or back of the shoulder, there may also be nausea, vomiting, and abdominal distention. A small number of persons may also experience slight jaundice. Chronic cholecystitis, on the other hand, manifests as frequent distress and distention in the upper abdomen, discomfort in the right upper abdomen which may refer to the right upper back, soreness, distention, and pain in the right upper back, poor appetite, a burning sensation in the stomach, belching, etc. These symptoms typically become more severe after eating greasy food, getting angry, mental stress, or catching cold.

In Chinese medicine, since there is pain, we know that the qi and blood are not flowing freely. However, in the case of cholecystitis and cholelithiasis, the main reason the qi and blood are not flowing freely is usually a combination of stuck or stagnant liver qi and damp heat. Damp heat, in turn, is mostly due to poor digestion, or what Chinese medicine refers to as spleen and stomach function. Therefore, in Chinese self-massage, most the manipulations recommended for cholecystitis and cholelithiasis either quicken the blood and move the qi in the areas that are painful or strengthen and regulate the spleen and stomach so as to transform and eliminate dampness and heat.

**Massage methods:**

1. Finger pressing tender points on the back: First, search by touch for tender points on the sides of the spine on the back. Then finger press and knead these tender points with the knuckles of both thumbs 100-200 times.

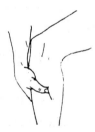

2. Pressing & kneading *Dan Nang* (M-LED-23): With the tips of both thumbs, search for tender points on the outsides of and just below the knees. Then press and knead these with strong force 100-200 times.

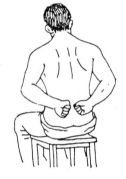

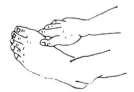

3. Pressing & kneading *Tai Chong* (Liv 3): With the tips of both thumbs, press and knead the points on the backs of the feet in the depression between the 1st and 2nd metatarsal 100-200 times.

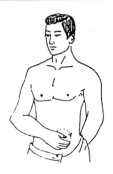

4. Circular rubbing the upper & middle abdomen: With one palm, circularly rub around the midpoint of the upper abdomen and the navel clockwise for 3-5 minutes each.

5. Obliquely rubbing the lateral costal regions: With both palms, rub both lateral costal regions from the armpits to the sides of the abdomen to and fro to produce a sensation of heat.

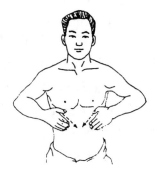

6. Pressing & kneading the points on the back:
With bent knuckles of both thumbs, press and knead the points *Ge Shu* (Bl 17, located 1.5 body inches lateral to the lower edge of the 7th thoracic vertebra), *Gan Shu* (Bl 18, located 1.5 body inches lateral to the lower edge of the 9th thoracic vertebra), and *Dan Shu* (Bl 19, located 1.5 body inches lateral to the lower edge of the 10th thoracic vertebra) approximately 100 times each. (See picture, page 92, #5)

7. Pressing & kneading *Yang Ling Quan* (GB 34):
With the tips of both thumbs, press and knead the points on the lateral sides of both knees in the depression in front of and below the small head of the fibula approximately 100 times each.

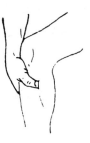

8. Pressing & kneading *Zu San Li* (St 36): With the tips of both thumbs, press and knead *Zu San Li* (located 3 body inches below the lower outside edge of the kneecap) approximately 100 times each. (See picture, page 88, #8)

When treating acute cholecystitis, first massage with strong force manipulations #1- 3 until the pain is relieved. Then go on to do manipulations #4-8. When treating chronic cholecystitis, the above manipulations should be done every day or every other day in the order given above. In that case, the force of the massage should be lighter. In addition, one should try to keep their peace of mind. Try not to become overly tense, over-excited, or over-fatigued. Get enough rest and avoid catching cold. Be careful about eating and drinking. Do not eat and drink too much at one meal, and eat less foods which are high in fat and protein. Form a good habit of regular bowel movements. And finally, do more exercises for strengthening the muscles of the back.

Acute attacks of gallbladder colic can often be relieved by acupuncture, while Chinese herbal medicine can actually dissolve gallstones and prevent acute attacks when taken regularly over a long period of time.

## O. Diabetes

Diabetes mellitus is a common endocrine disease in developed countries where there is plenty of sugar and sweets as well as fatty, oily foods and excessive protein. It is characterized by the so-called three polys — polydipsia (frequent drinking), polyphagia (frequent eating), and polyuria (frequent urination). In addition, there is often obesity at first then becoming emaciation and the urine has a sweet taste due to the presence of sugar. From the Western medical point of view, diabetes is caused by either an absolute or relative inadequacy of insulin. Therefore, the body is incapable of metabolizing fat, protein, and sugars properly. This then causes a secondary disturbance of water and electrolytes.

Although proper regulation of the diet is absolutely necessary in controlling and reversing diabetes, Chinese self-massage can also help relieve its symptoms, prevent the disease from worsening, and regulate the internal functions of the body. In Chinese medicine, diabetes is related to heat in the lungs and/or stomach with weakness of the lungs, spleen, and/or kidneys. Therefore, Chinese self-massage maneuvers for diabetes mainly aim at supplementing and regulating the function of the lungs, spleen, stomach, and kidneys and clearing or eliminating pathological heat from the body.

**Massage methods:**

1. Pressing & kneading *Zhong Wan* (CV 12), *Liang Men* (St 21), and *Jian Li* (CV 11): With the tip of one or both middle fingers, press and knead *Zhong Wan* (the midpoint of the upper abdomen), *Liang Men* (located 2 body inches lateral to *Zhong Wan*), and *Jian Li* (located 1 body inch below *Zhong Wan*) approximately 100 times each.

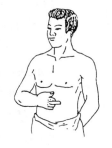

2. Circular rubbing the abdomen: With one palm, circularly rub the abdomen around the navel counterclockwise approximately 200 times.

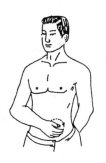

3. Straight pushing the abdomen: Place both palms on both sides of the abdomen. Push downward straight 30-50 times.

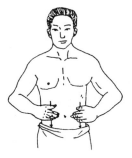

4. Pressing & kneading the points on the back: With the bent knuckles of both thumbs, press and knead the points *Fei Shu* (Bl 13, located 1.5 body inches lateral to the lower edge of the

3rd thoracic vertebra), *Pi Shu* (Bl 20, located 1.5 body inches lateral to the lower edge of the 11th thoracic vertebra), *Wei Shu* (Bl 21, located 1.5 body inches lateral to the lower edge of the 12th thoracic vertebra), *Shen Shu* (Bl 23, located 1.5 body inches lateral to the lower edge of the 2nd lumbar vertebra), and *Yang Gang* (Bl 48, located 1.5 body inches lateral to the lower edge of the 3rd lumbar vertebra) approximately 100 times each. (See picture, page 92, #5)

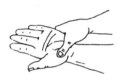

5. Pressing & kneading *Yu Ji* (Lu 10): With the thumb of the right hand, press and knead the left *Yu Ji* (the midpoint between the base of the thumb and the base of the palm on the lateral side of the palm) 30-50 times. Then repeat this procedure on the right *Yu Ji*.

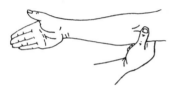

6. Pressing & kneading *Qu Ze* (Per 3): With the tip of the middle finger of the right hand, press and knead the left *Qu Ze* (located at the ulnar side of the tendon in the transverse elbow crease) 30-50 times. The repeat this procedure on the right *Qu Ze*.

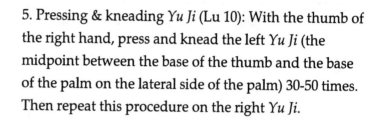

7. Pressing & kneading *Zu San Li* (St 36): With the tips of both thumbs, press and knead *Zu San Li* (located 3 body inches below the lower outside edge of the kneecap) approximately 100 times each.

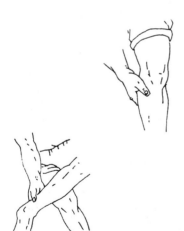

8. Pressing & kneading *San Yin Jiao* (Sp 6): With the tips of both thumbs, press and knead the points located 3 body inches above the tip of the inner ankles 50-100 times each side.

Self-massage alone cannot cure or control diabetes if not supported by a clear, bland diet. One should eat more vegetables and bean products like tofu and tempeh, eat less in general, and eat less greasy, fried, fatty, sweet, sugary, or acrid, spicy foods. One should also avoid alcohol. One can eat a certain amount of lean meat. Try to exercise regularly, adjust work and rest harmoniously, do not worry too much, and adjust your sexual life and reduce the frequency of sexual intercourse. In addition, Chinese herbal medicine can definitely help treat and control diabetes mellitus.

CHAPTER
6

# Chinese Self-massage for the Treatment of Gynecological Diseases

## 1. Irregular menstruation

Normally, menstruation in women occurs once a month or every 28-30 days. In Chinese medicine, the menses also fall within the normal range if they come 3-5 days earlier or later than 28-30 days. Typically, the menses last 3-7 days and their amount is generally 50-80 ml. In most cases, the color of the menstruate is dark red without any blood clots. There may be, however, small fragments of endometrium. The consistency of the menstruate is neither thick nor thin and it is without any especially bad smell. Irregular menstruation means that the cycle and/or the amount and color of the menses is abnormal yet without any organic disease of the reproductive system. Irregular menstruation is a generic term which includes several different menstrual diseases according to Chinese medicine. These are early menstruation, delayed menstruation, erratic menstruation, excessive menstruation, and scanty menstruation.

According to Chinese medicine, all irregular menstruation can be divided into two broad patterns. These are called vacuity and repletion. Vacuity means that some viscera or organ in the body is hypofunctioning or not doing its proper job *vis a vis* menstruation. In this case, treatment aims at supplementing the viscera which is hypofunctioning. Repletion means that some organ or some pathological qi or energy in the body is excessive. This repletion or excess either causes the viscera in charge of menstruation to malfunction or causes erratic or hindered flow of the qi and blood. In that case, treatment aims at eliminating or clearing the pathological qi from the body and restoring the free and easy flow of qi and blood. The main viscera in charge of menstruation are the three viscera in charge of manufacturing then blood — the heart, spleen, and kidneys — and the three viscera in charge of controlling the blood — the heart, spleen, and liver.

In general, the symptoms of the vacuity pattern are a lighter than normal colored menstruate which also tends to be thinner than normal in consistency, fatigue, bodily weakness, heart palpitations, shortness of breath, dizziness, poor appetite, low back and knee soreness and weakness, and a pale facial complexion. The typical symptoms of the repletion pattern are a deep red or purplish red, thicker than normal menstruate which contains blood clots and is accompanied by vexation, irritability, lower abdominal distention and pain which refuses pressure, and breast distention and pain.

When treating irregular menstruation with Chinese self-massage, one should differentiate between these vacuity and repletion patterns. Generally, self-massage should be done once a day beginning 1 week before the onset of menstruation until menses begin to flow freely. In vacuity cases, self-massage may also be done after the menstruation as well.

**Massage methods:**

1. Pressing & kneading *Zhong Wan* (CV 12), *Qi Hai* (CV 6), and *Guan Yuan* (CV 4): With one palm, press and knead the midpoint of the upper abdomen, the point 1.5 body inches below the navel, and the midpoint of the lower abdomen approximately 100 times each.

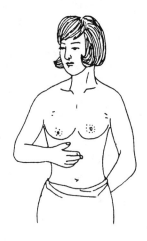

2. Pressing & kneading the points on the back: With the bent knuckles of both thumbs, press and knead the points *Fei Shu* (Bl 13, located 1.5 body inches lateral to the lower edge of the 3rd thoracic vertebra), *Xin Shu* (Bl 15, located 1.5 body inches lateral to the lower edge of the 5th thoracic vertebra), *Gan Shu* (Bl 18, located 1.5 body inches lateral to the lower edge of the 9th thoracic vertebra), *Pi Shu* (Bl 20, located 1.5 body inches lateral to the lower edge of the 11th thoracic vertebra), *Shen Shu* (Bl 23, located 1.5 body inches lateral to the lower edge of the 2nd lumbar vertebra), and *Guan Yuan Shu* (Bl 26, located 1.5 body inches lateral to the lower edge of the 5th lumbar vertebra) approximately 100 times each. (See picture, page 92, #5)

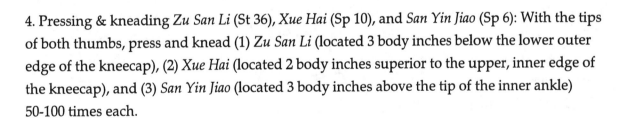

3. Pressing & kneading *Ba Liao* (Bl 31-34): With the bent knuckles of both thumbs, press and knead the eight posterior sacral foramina pair by pair starting with the highest ones 30-50 times each.

4. Pressing & kneading *Zu San Li* (St 36), *Xue Hai* (Sp 10), and *San Yin Jiao* (Sp 6): With the tips of both thumbs, press and knead (1) *Zu San Li* (located 3 body inches below the lower outer edge of the kneecap), (2) *Xue Hai* (located 2 body inches superior to the upper, inner edge of the kneecap), and (3) *San Yin Jiao* (located 3 body inches above the tip of the inner ankle) 50-100 times each.

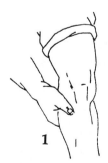
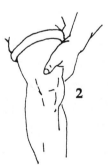
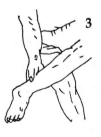

5. Rubbing & patting the lumbosacral region:
This manipulation is specifically for the vacuity
pattern. With one palm, rub the lumbosacral
area transversely to and fro until there is a
sensation of heat. Then, with the hollow palm,
pat the area with gentle force 30-50 times.

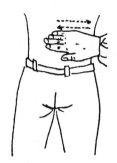

6. Rubbing the lateral costal
regions & lower abdomen:
This manipulation is specifically
for the repletion pattern. With
the two palms, rub obliquely
from the armpits to the midpoint
of the upper abdomen to and
fro to produce a sensation of
heat. Then rub from the lower
edges of the ribcage to the
midpoint of the lower abdomen
to produce a sensation of heat.
Finally, push with one palm
from the navel to the midpoint
of the pubic bone 5-10 times.

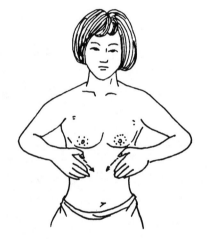

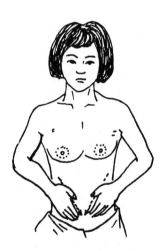

When treating the vacuity pattern, the force of the massage should be light, while when
treating the repletion pattern, the force should be relatively heavy. Most Western women
with menstrual irregularity actually have a combination of the repletion and vacuity
patterns. In such cases, the force should be heavy before the onset of menstruation and the
force should be light after the menses have ceased. In general, women with menstrual
irregularity should eat a clear, bland diet, get regular aerobic exercise at least 3-4 times each
week, and practice deep relaxation for 20 minutes every day. In particular, women should

not exercise too heavily or become over-fatigued during menstruation, nor should they eat cold, raw, chilled, or frozen foods during and right before menstruation. For women 35 years old and older, the likelihood of suffering from a combined vacuity and repletion pattern is even greater. In such cases, Chinese herbal medicine prescribed by a professional practitioner trained in Chinese medical gynecology is extremely helpful. In general, professional acupuncturists or practitioners of Chinese medicine can help women decide if their condition is one of repletion or vacuity and can give many more tips on how to treat irregular menstruation based on the individual woman's personal pattern and needs. Gynecology is one of Chinese medicine's most effective specialties.

## 2. Dysmenorrhea

Dysmenorrhea refers to lower abdominal, low back, or even thigh pain either before, during, or after menstruation. This pain may be mild or extremely severe. It may consist of generalized cramping or very localized sharp, stabbing pain. If the pain is very severe, it may be accompanied by dripping cold sweat from the head and face, cold hands and feet, nausea, and vomiting. It is normal if a woman experiences slight distention and pain in the lower abdomen and low back before or after menstruation as long as this does not affect her normal work or study or need treatment for relief. However, if period pain is anything more than this, it should be treated, either by oneself or a professional health care practitioner. Some women think that their periods are naturally painful, that this is a woman's lot. However, in Chinese medicine, this is not so.

Remember, the cardinal statement about pain in Chinese medicine is, "If there is pain, there is no free flow." Therefore, the Chinese self-massage maneuvers given below mainly aim at restoring and promoting the smooth and free flow of the qi and blood to and through the pelvis. If the qi and blood in the pelvis flow freely and without obstruction, there will be no pain.

Chinese self-massage for treating dysmenorrhea should be begun 1 week before the onset of menstruation and continued once per day until the menses begin. This is considered one course of treatment. The next course should then be begun again 1 week before the next menstruation. Primary dysmenorrhea, meaning dysmenorrhea which begins with menarche and is not associated with any organic disease, can generally be cured or relieved after 3-6 courses of treatment. For acquired dysmenorrhea, meaning painful periods associated with some other organic disease such as pelvic inflammation or endometriosis, the primary disease should be treated first and, as the primary disease is cured, the dysmenorrhea will disappear. Acupuncture and Chinese herbal medicine are good choices for the treatment of even organic gynecological diseases associated with dysmenorrhea. At the time of menstruation, self-massage should not be done on the abdomen and low back. However, it can be done on the extremities on points which can relieve pelvic pain.

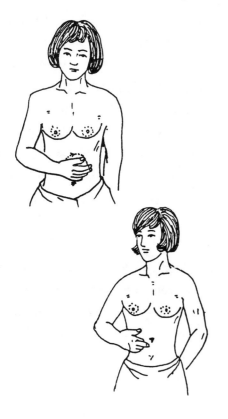

**Massage methods:**

1. Circular rubbing the abdomen & *Guan Yuan* (CV 4): With one palm, circularly rub the abdomen around the navel and around the midpoint of the lower abdomen clockwise for 3-5 minutes each.

2. Finger pressing the points on the lower abdomen: With the tip of one thumb or middle finger, press the points *Qi Hai* (CV 6, located 1.5 body inches below the navel), *Guan Yuan* (CV 4, located 3 body inches below the navel), *Zhong Ji* (CV 3, located 4 body inches below the navel), and *Gui Lai* (St 29, located 2 body inches lateral to *Zhong Ji*) 30-50 times each.

3. Pushing the lower abdomen: With one palm, push the lower abdomen from the navel to the midpoint of the lower edge of the abdomen 30-50 times.

4. Pressing & kneading *Shen Shu* (Bl 23) & *Ba Liao* (Bl 31-34): With the bent knuckles of both thumbs, press and knead the points which are 1.5 body inches lateral to the 2nd lumbar vertebra and the eight posterior sacral foramina 30-50 times each.

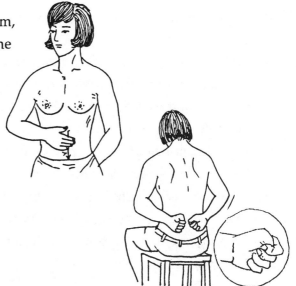

5. Transversely rubbing the lumbosacral region: With one palm, transversely rub the lumbosacral area to and fro to produce a sensation of heat. (See picture, page 108, #5)

6. Pressing & kneading *San Yin Jiao* (Sp 6): With the tips of both thumbs, press and knead the points which are 3 body inches above the tip of the inner ankles of both legs 100-200 times. (See picture, page 102, #8)

7. Grasping & kneading *Xue Hai* (Sp 10): Place the pads of both thumbs on *Xue Hai* (located 2 body inches above the inner, upper edge of the kneecap) of both legs. Grasp the points strongly 3-5 times and then knead them 30-50 times. (See page 107, item #4, picture #2)

The same general advice on diet and lifestyle given above for irregular menstruation should also be followed for painful menstruation. In addition, do not swim or bathe in cold water during menstruation or engage in sexual intercourse during menstruation.

## 3. Amenorrhea

Amenorrhea means absence of menstruation. A woman may be diagnosed as suffering from amenorrhea if she is over 18 years of age and has never had a period or if a woman after menarche does not have their menses for more than three consecutive months. The first condition is referred to as primary amenorrhea and the second is called secondary amenorrhea. Amenorrhea does not include cessation of menstruation during pregnancy which is normal. In modern Western medicine, there are many causes of amenorrhea which are divided into functional and organic types. Chinese self-massage is very effective for treating functional amenorrhea. Self-massage is not effective for treating a number of types of organic amenorrhea, such as congenital absence of the uterus, ovaries, or vagina and congenital imperforate hymen.

In Chinese medicine, amenorrhea is usually due either to hypofunctioning of the viscera which manufactures the blood — the heart, spleen, and kidneys — or to lack of free flow of the qi and blood to and through the pelvis. Therefore, Chinese self-massage for amenorrhea is mainly aimed at improving the function of those viscera which create and control the blood and improving and regulating the flow of qi and blood to and through the pelvis and uterus.

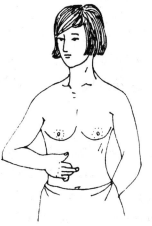

**Massage methods:**

1. Pressing & kneading *Zhong Wan* (CV 12), *Qi Hai* (CV 6), and *Guan Yuan* (CV 4): With the tip of one middle finger, press and knead the midpoint of the upper abdomen, the point located 1.5 body inches below the navel, and the midpoint of the lower abdomen 100-200 times each.

2. Circular rubbing *Guan Yuan* (CV 4): With one palm, circularly rub the lower abdomen around the midpoint of the lower abdomen for 5-10 minutes.

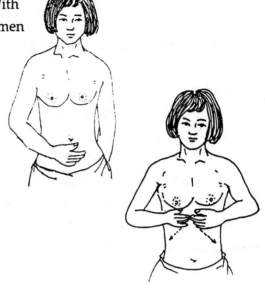

3. Pushing apart the abdomen: With the index and middle fingers of both hands, push apart the abdomen from the midpoint of the upper abdomen obliquely to the sides of the abdomen approximately 100 times.

4. Rubbing the lateral costal regions & the sides of the lower abdomen: With both palms, rub the lateral costal regions from the armpits obliquely to the upper abdomen to and fro to produce a sensation of heat. Then rub the sides of the lower abdomen from the bottom of the ribcage to the midpoint of the lower abdomen to and fro to produce a sensation of heat.

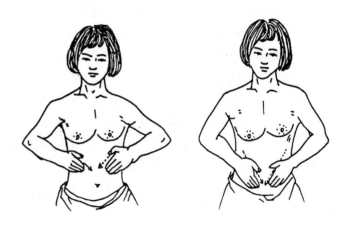

5. Pressing & kneading the points on the back: With the bent knuckles of both thumbs, press and knead the points *Gan Shu* (Bl 18, located 1.5 body inches lateral to the lower edge of the 9th thoracic vertebra), *Pi Shu* (Bl 20, located 1.5 body inches lateral to the lower edge of the 11th thoracic vertebra), *Shen Shu* (Bl 23, located 1.5 body inches lateral to the lower edge of the 2nd lumbar vertebra), and *Ba Liao* (Bl 31-34, located over the eight sacral foramina)

approximately 100 times each. Then, with the bent knuckles of one thumb, press and knead *Ming Men* (GV 4, located just below the 2nd lumbar vertebra) and *Yao Yang Guan* (GV 3, located just below the 4th lumbar vertebra) approximately 100 times each. (See picture, page 92, #5)

6. Transversely rubbing the lumbosacral region: With one palm, transversely rub the lumbosacral region to and fro to produce a sensation of heat. (See picture, page 108, #5)

7. Pressing & kneading *Zu San Li* (St 36), *Xue Hai* (Sp 10), and *San Yin Jiao* (Sp 6): With the tips of both thumbs, press and knead *Zu San Li* (located 3 body inches below the lower, outside edge of the kneecap), *Xue Hai* (located 2 body inches above the upper, inner edge of the kneecap), and *San Yin Jiao* (located 3 body inches above the tip of the inner ankle) approximately 100 times each. (See picture, page 107, #4)

In the West, one of the common causes of amenorrhea is low body fat in turn due to over-exercising and insufficient eating. Although women whose qi and blood are not freely flowing need more exercise in order to promote the free and easy flow of the qi and blood, women who are too thin to have a period may actually have to exercise less and eat more. In addition, in the West, some women suffer from scanty periods and amenorrhea due to the adoption of a strict vegetarian diet. Although Chinese medicine does not recommend eating a lot of meat, some animal protein is necessary for many women living in a temperate climate whose bodies and metabolism were formed on meat and who lead very active work lives. In such cases, adding a *little* meat to the diet can be very beneficial.

## 4. Pelvic inflammatory disease

Pelvic inflammatory disease (PID) refers to the inflammation of the internal reproductive organs in a woman. This may include the uterus, fallopian tubes, ovaries, and surrounding pelvic tissues. Such inflammation may be located at one area only or may occur in several areas at the same time. It is called salpingitis if the inflammation is located only in the fallopian tubes and ovaritis if it is located only in the ovaries.

116

Pelvic inflammatory disease can also be divided into acute and chronic types. Acute pelvic inflammatory disease is accompanied by severe symptoms. It is caused by the complications of childbirth, postpartum complications, abortion, uterine curettage (*i.e.*, D & C), poor sterilization and antiseptic procedures when putting in or removing an intrauterine device (IUD), or ascending infection contracted during sexual intercourse or while bathing during menstruation. Acute PID may also be a secondary disease due to infection of other organs in the abdominal cavity.

Chronic pelvic inflammation is, in most cases, caused by improper treatment of acute pelvic inflammation or due to the prolonged existence of acute PID. However, in some cases, the patient may have no history of acute PID. Chronic PID is a common gynecological disease. It is recalcitrant to treatment and easily relapses. Patients with chronic PID generally have no obvious generalized symptoms. Some of them may have mild fever. The main symptoms of chronic PID are a vague pain or sagging discomfort in the lower abdomen and an aching pain in the lumbosacral region which typically gets worse during menstruation, at ovulation, when the woman is tired, or after sexual intercourse. Other symptoms, such as fatigue, listlessness, insomnia, profuse leukorrhea, and irregular menstruation, may be present at other times. Infertility may also be caused by PID. There is tenderness in the sides of the lower abdomen, and there may be some ropey matter palpable on the sides of the lower abdomen in prolonged cases.

Chinese self-massage is very effective for treating chronic PID. Acute PID or an acute attack of chronic pelvic inflammation may be treated with self-massage after first being treated with internal medicine, be that Western antibiotics or Chinese herbal medicine, and after the acute inflammation has been controlled. Chinese self-massage for PID mainly aims at improving the flow of qi and blood through the pelvis. Since it is said in Chinese medicine that, "Enduring diseases damage the kidneys", there are also manuevers meant to supplement the kidneys for chronic PID.

**Massage methods:**

1. Pressing & kneading *Qi Hai* (CV 6), *Guan Yuan* (CV 4), and *Zhong Ji* (CV 3): With the base of one palm, press and knead the point 1.5 body inches below the navel, the mid-point of the lower abdomen, and the point 4 body inches below the navel 100-200 times each to produce a hot sensation in the abdomen.

2. Pressing & kneading *Zi Gong* (M-CA-18) and tender points: With both thumbs, press and knead *Zi Gong* (located 3 body inches lateral to the point 4 body inches below the navel) approximately 100 times. Then press and knead any tender points around *Zi Gong* to produce a sensation of soreness and distention. If cordlike or ropey tissue is felt, press and knead these in the same way.

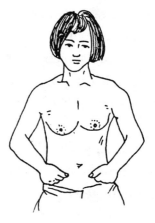

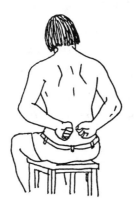

3. Pressing & kneading *Shen Shu* (Bl 23) and *Ba Liao* (Bl 31-34): With the bent knuckles of both thumbs, press and knead the points which are 1.5 body inches lateral to the lower edge of the 2nd lumbar vertebra and the eight sacral foramina approximately 100 times each.

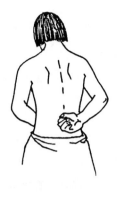

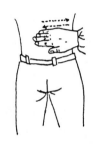

4. Pounding the lumbosacral region: With the back of one fist, lightly pound the lumbosacral region 30-50 times.

5. Transversely rubbing the lumbosacral region: With one palm, transversely rub the lumbosacral area to and fro to produce a sensation of heat.

6. Pressing & kneading *Xue Hai* (Sp 10) and *San Yin Jiao* (Sp 6): With the tips of both thumbs, press and knead *Xue Hai* (located 2 body inches above the upper, inner edge of the kneecap) and *San Yin Jiao* (located 3 body inches above the tip of the inner ankle) approximately 100 times each. (See page 107, item #4, pictures #2 & 3)

7. Rubbing the medial sides of the legs: With one palm, rub the inner side of the thigh up and down and the inner side of the lower leg up and down to produce a sensation of heat. Then rub the other leg in the same way. ➡

Although antibiotics are effective for bringing an episode of acute PID under control, they are not effective for chronic PID or repeated flare-ups of PID. In those cases, acupuncture and Chinese herbal medicine are much more effective since they take the entire pattern of the patient into account. In chronic conditions, the infection, if there is one, is not as important as the host's immune system, and Chinese medicine can most definitely strengthen immunity and thus allow the individual herself to combat the infection or inflammation. In chronic PID, it is very important to get

**119**

adequate exercise, to improve one's coping skills through daily deep relaxation if there is family or job stress, and to eat a clear, bland diet.

## 5. Abnormal vaginal discharge

Every adult woman should have a certain amount of vaginal secretion in order to lubricate and protect the membranes of the vagina. However, in some women, these vaginal secretions may become excessive and they may also change their color, consistency, and become malodorous. Such abnormal vaginal secretions are called abnormal vaginal discharge in Chinese medicine and are one of the four main groups of gynecological disease in Chinese medicine. Abnormal vaginal discharge can be caused by many gynecological diseases, such as yeast and trichomoniasis infections, and there are a number of different patterns described in the Chinese medical literature. However, all these patterns involve a more than normal discharge of fluids from the vagina. In Chinese medicine, such abnormal fluids are associated with dampness and phlegm. Therefore, Chinese self-massage seeks to treat abnormal vaginal discharge by strengthening and regulating the two main viscera in charge of body fluids — the spleen and kidneys — and by regulating and promoting the flow of qi and blood through the pelvis and genitalia.

**Massage methods:**

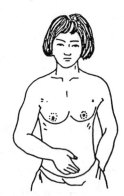

1. Kneading the lower abdomen: With the heel of one palm, knead the midpoint of the lower abdomen with weak or medium force for 3-5 minutes.

2. Rubbing the sides of the lower abdomen: With both palms, rub the sides of the lower abdomen to and fro from the base of the ribcage to the midpoint of the lower abdomen until there is a sensation of heat. (See picture, page 113, #4)

3. Pressing & kneading *Gui Lai* (St 29) and *Dai Mai* (GB 26): With the tips of both middle fingers, press and knead *Gui Lai* (located 2 body inches lateral to the point 4 body inches below the navel) and *Dai Mai* (located below the armpits and at the level of the navel) approximately 100 times each. The force of these manipulations should be strong.

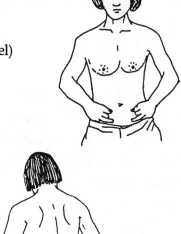

4. Pressing & kneading *Shen Shu* (Bl 23) and *Pang Guang Shu* (Bl 28): With the bent knuckles of both thumbs, press and knead the points which are 1.5 body inches lateral to the lower edge of the 2nd lumbar vertebra and 1.5 body inches lateral to the 2nd sacral vertebra approximately 100 times each.

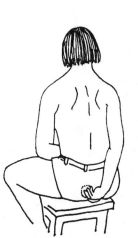

5. Transversely rubbing the lumbosacral region: With one palm, transversely rub the lumbosacral region to and fro to produce a sensation of heat. (See picture, page 117, #5)

6. Kneading *Chang Qiang* (GV 1): With the tip of one middle finger, knead the point located 0.5 body inches below the tip of the tailbone approximately 100 times.

7. Rubbing the medial sides of the thighs: With one palm, rub the inner side of the thigh up and down to produce a sensation of heat. Then rub the other thigh in the same way. (See picture, page 117, #7)

8. Pressing & kneading *Zu San Li* (St 36), *Feng Long* (St 40), *Xue Hai* (Sp 10), and *San Yin Jiao* (Sp 6): With the tips of both thumbs, press and knead (1) *Zu San Li* (located 3 body inches below the lower outside edge of the kneecap), (2) *Feng Long* (located 8 body inches above the tip of the outer ankle), (3) *Xue Hai* (located 2 body inches above the outer, upper edge of the kneecap), and (4) *San Yin Jiao* (located 3 body inches above the tip of the inner ankle) approximately 100 times each.

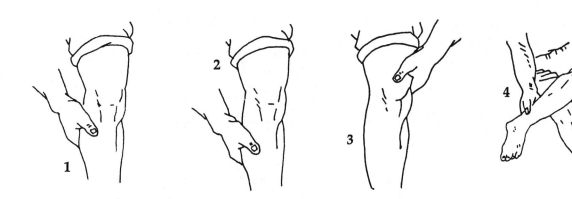

Women with chronic excessive vaginal discharge with external vaginal itching and irritation should eat a clear, bland diet and stay away from sugars and sweets, anything that molds easily, like strawberries, cheese, and bread, or anything made through fermentation, such as cheese, bread, alcohol, or vinegar. If the discharge is thick and curdy or thick and yellowish, one can try filling a #0 gelatin capsule with boric acid available from neighborhood pharmacies. Insert one of these each evening before bed as a vaginal suppository. Other potential home treatments are douching with either vinegar or acidophilus yogurt. In addition, acupuncture and Chinese herbal medicine are both usually effective for the common diseases which cause or are associated with abnormal vaginal discharge. However, one should immediately see a Western MD if there is a multicolored vaginal discharge, sometimes white, sometimes red and bloody, and sometimes yellow and green as if mixed with purulent pus, since this may be a sign of cervical cancer.

## 6. Mastitis

Mastitis is mostly seen in breast-feeding women and especially in primiparas or first time mothers. It typically occurs 1 month after childbirth. Most commonly, there is distention, swelling, or a lump with redness and pain above the nipple in one breast. This may be accompanied by high fever or no fever depending on the cause. If left untreated, such an infection of the breast may become a purulent breast abscess. According to modern Western medicine, mastitis is most often due to a *Staphylococcus aureus* infection invading the milk ducts and lymphatic vessels. In Chinese medicine, mastitis may be due to any combination of three causes: 1) infection from outside, 2) over-eating postpartum and especially over-eating hot, spicy, greasy, fried, fatty foods and/or drinking alcohol, and 3) emotional stress. In any of these cases, heat accumulates in the breast obstructing and blocking the free flow of qi and blood through the breasts. Thus there is pain, swelling, and redness. Based on this, Chinese self-massage treats mastitis mostly by promoting the flow of qi and blood through the breasts.

**Massage methods:**

1. Pushing & kneading *Shan Zhong* (CV 17): With the tip of one middle finger, press and knead the point in the middle of the chest on the sternum at the same level as the 4th intercostal space or between where the nipples would be in a man 100-200 times to produce a sensation of soreness and distention. Then, with the lateral sides of both thumbs, push apart from this point to both sides 30-50 times.

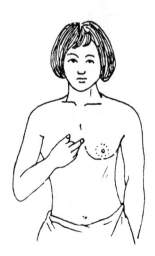

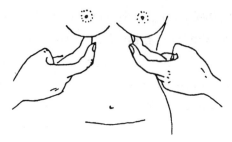

2. Pressing & kneading *Ru Gen* (St 18): With the tips of both middle fingers, press and knead the points 1 body inch below each nipple 50-100 times to produce a sensation of soreness and distention.

3. Pushing & kneading the breast: With one palm, push the breast with a weak force from every side of the breast towards the nipple and then circularly rub and knead the breast for approximately 5 minutes. The force should become gradually stronger as the rubbing and kneading continue.

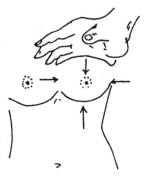

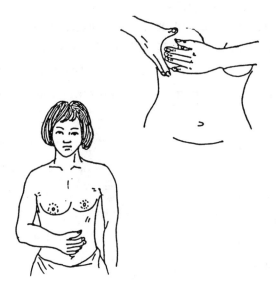

4. Squeezing out static milk: With the thumb and index finger of one hand, hold the nipple and squeeze out the milk with weak force for several minutes to remove any stagnant milk within the ducts.

5. Circular rubbing the abdomen: With one palm, circularly rub the abdomen around the navel clockwise for approximately 5 minutes.

6. Pressing & kneading the points on the back: With the bent knuckles of both thumbs, press and knead the points *Gan Shu* (Bl 18, located 1.5 body inches lateral to the lower edge of the 9th thoracic vertebra), *Pi Shu* (Bl 20, located 1.5 body inches lateral to the lower edge of the

11th thoracic vertebra), and *Wei Shu* (Bl 21, located 1.5 body inches lateral to the lower edge of the 12th thoracic vertebra) approximately 100 times each. (See picture, page 92, #5)

In the West, mastitis *un*accompanied by fever, chills, and other signs of external infection is usually due to emotional stress and frustration. However, this can be complicated by eating hot, spicy or greasy, fatty foods. In such cases, it is important for the woman to eat a clear, bland diet and to try to relax and calm her mind. Besides the Chinese self-massage manuevers given above, it will be helpful to use a warm, ginger compress over the affected breast when breast-feeding. This is made by simmering several slices of fresh ginger in water for 5-7 minutes. Then immerse a towel or cloth in this "ginger tea", wring it out, and apply while still hot over the area of pain and inflammation. Keep this in place for 10-15 minutes each time, dipping the cloth again into the hot ginger tea as the cloth cools off. If done while breast-feeding, this will help expel any stagnant milk in the ducts and dissipate the inflammation. Prior to birth, the mother should condition her nipples by pulling on them and also rubbing them with a coarse cloth. *Chinese Medicinal Teas* by Zong & Liscum, Blue Poppy Press, gives a number of simple Chinese herbal remedies for mastitis.

## 7. Fibrocystic breast disease

Among many Western practitioners, there is some controversy over whether so-called fibrocystic breast disease (FBD) is actually a disease. Some clinicians regard it as merely a symptom of aging. It refers to increased growth of fibrous and/or cystic tissue in the female breast. It is often seen among women 25-45 years old. Typically, this condition gets worse with age but remits after menopause. Often it is associated with premenstrual breast distention and pain. Commonly, cystic lumps in the breast grow during the premenstruum and may become sore to the touch. After menstruation, these lumps recede in size and number and become painless. There is no change in the color or shape of the skin over the breasts, nor is there any change in the nipples. Although this disease is considered benign, there is an increased statistical incidence of breast cancer in women with FBD. This is interesting since Western researchers and clinicians are now beginning to regard breast cancer as a disease of aging in women the same way that prostate cancer is a disease of aging in men.

In Chinese medicine, the breasts are connected to the liver. It is the liver which is in charge of keeping the qi in the body freely and easily flowing. The liver is also called the temperamental organ. Its function of maintaining the free flow of the qi is easily negatively affected by emotional stress, anger, and frustration. For almost 1,000 years, Chinese doctors have attributed the occurrence of premenstrual breast distention and pain, FBD, and breast cancer primarily to emotional stress. Stress, anger, and frustration result in the liver becoming depressed and qi flow stagnant. Since the liver is connected to the breasts, if the liver qi becomes stagnant and depressed, the flow of qi in the breast as well as the blood pushed by the qi may also become stagnant in the breasts. This then leads to pain and the formation of lumps. Therefore, the Chinese self-massage manuevers for treating FBD are mainly aimed at improving the flow of qi and blood in the breasts and also in the Chinese medical concept of the liver. The self-massage regimen below may also be used to treat benign breast lumps.

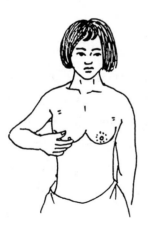

**Massage methods:**

1. Lightly kneading the lumps: Press any lumpy area from both sides with the thumb and index finger of one hand and knead with weak force. Then lightly knead the entire breast for approximately 10 minutes. Knead both breasts with both palms if there are lumps in both breasts.

2. Pressing & kneading *Shan Zhong* (CV 17): With the tip of one middle finger, press and knead the point in the middle of the chest level with the 4th intercostal space 100-200 times.

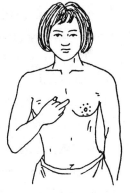
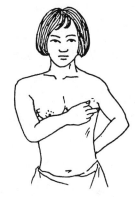

3. Kneading the underarms: With the tips of both middle fingers, lightly knead the area under the armpits 100-200 times.

4. Pushing the breasts: With both palms, lightly push both breasts from every side of the breasts to the nipples for 3-5 minutes. (See picture, page 122, #3)

5. Rubbing the lateral costal regions: With both palms, rub both lateral costal regions from the armpits to the sides of the abdomen for 3-5 minutes. (See picture, page 113, #4)

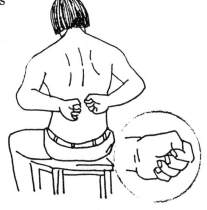

6. Pressing & kneading *Gan Shu* (Bl 18): With the bent knuckles of both thumbs, press and knead the points which are 1.5 body inches lateral to the lower edge of the 9th thoracic vertebra 100-200 times.

Because fibrocystic breasts and premenstrual breast distention and pain are so closely associated with mental-emotional stress, it is very important for women with breast disease to practice daily deep relaxation. Because these conditions are also associated with blood stasis and qi stagnation, it is very important for women with these conditions to get adequate, preferably aerobic exercise in order to move the qi which pushes the blood. Deep relaxation and maintaining a free and easy affect gets at the root of the problem, while regular exercise keeps any stagnant qi from accumulating too badly. Since many women with breast conditions also suffer from menstrual irregularity of one sort or another, both of these conditions should be treated at the same time since they are interrelated. In women in their 40s, some Chinese herbal medicine to strengthen the spleen and supplement the kidneys can usually speed up the healing process.

# Traumatology Department Diseases

## 1. Stiff neck

Stiff neck or torticollis mainly manifests as pain, rigidity, and spasm of the neck and back of the neck and limitation of neck movement. In most cases, it is caused by the hyperextension of the muscles in the neck and nuchal region on one side due to improper pillow height or by muscular spasm due to exposure to cold of the back of the neck while sleeping. Therefore, in most cases, it is experienced in the morning when getting up. Mild cases may recover by themselves within 1-2 days, while severe cases accompanied by severe pain in the head, upper back, and/or shoulder may last for several weeks. There is marked tenderness and muscular spasm on the affected side of the neck.

Chinese self-massage is very effective for treating cases of stiff neck with light symptoms. If there is severe pain and severe limitation of neck movement, acupuncture or professionally administered Chinese medical massage should be used. If a tender point is found in the middle of the nape of the neck and is accompanied by numbness of the arm and fingers, this suggests a problem with one of the cervical vertebra and the patient should definitely see a professional health care practitioner.

In Chinese medicine, this and most other types of musculoskeletal pain are called *bi* conditions. *Bi* means blockage. In addition, because there is pain, we know that the qi and blood are not flowing freely in the affected area. Therefore, Chinese self-massage for this condition is primarily aimed at restoring and promoting the free and smooth flow of qi and blood in the local area.

**Massage methods:**

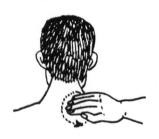

1. Kneading & circular rubbing the neck and nape: With one palm, knead and circularly rub the affected side of the neck and nape of the neck from the base of the skull to the upper back. Then turn the head towards the shoulder on the affected side until there is a feeling of heat, comfort is attained in the local area, and the pain is relieved.

2. Grasping the nape: With the thumb, index, and middle fingers of one hand, grasp the muscles of the nape of the neck on the affected side from the base of the skull to the shoulder several times.

3. Rubbing the nape: With one palm, rub the nape of the neck on the affected side from the base of the skull to the upper back and shoulder until there is a feeling of heat.

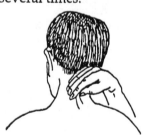

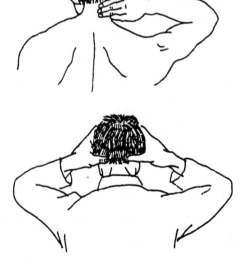

4. Pressing & kneading *Feng Chi* (GB 20): With the tips of both thumbs, press and knead the points just slightly above the posterior hairline and in the depression between the mastoid process and the long muscles at the back of the neck 30-50 times. Also rotate the head while kneading.

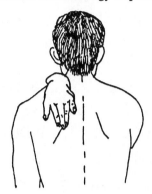

5. Pressing & kneading *Tian Zong* (SI 11): With the tip of the middle finger, press and knead the point in the center of the scapula below its spine 100-200 times to produce a feeling of soreness and distention in the upper back. At the same time, rotate the head slowly, starting out with small circles and expanding to larger circles. A relaxed feeling should be felt in the neck.

6. Pressing & kneading the tender points: With the tip of one thumb, press and knead any tender points on the neck, beginning with weak pressure and gradually increasing to strong. Then pluck the point for approximately 2-3 minutes.

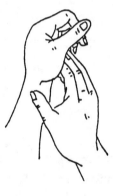

7. Nipping & kneading *Hou Xi* (SI 3) and *Lie Que* (Lu 7): With the nail and tip of the thumb, nip and knead *Hou Xi* (located on the ulnar edge of the palm, just behind the knuckle under the little finger on the palmar surface of the hand) and *Lie Que* (located 1.5 body inches above the transverse crease of the wrist on the lateral side of the forearm) 50-100 times for each point on each side. This maneuver is most effective if a feeling of soreness and distention at the points or radiating to the upper arm is felt.

8. Pressing & kneading *Luo Zhen* (M-UE-24): With the tip of the thumb, press and knead the point located 0.5 body inches behind the base of the index and middle fingers on the back of the hand on the affected side approximately 100 times. This point is called Crick in the Neck Point.

9. Hot compress: Put a towel in hot water, wring it out, and place it as a compress on the neck. As the towel cools, repeat this several times. Afterwards, a massage ointment, such as

Tiger Balm, Temple of Heaven, or Po Som An Oil (*Bao Xin An You*) may be applied on the neck while massaging into the affected side.

Chinese self-massage is usually effective for stiff neck, affecting a cure in 2-3 treatments. Those who often have a stiff neck should constantly massage on their neck and shoulders and combine this with rhythmical movement of the neck in order to prevent cervical spondylopathy.

## 2. Cervical spondylopathy

Cervical spondylopathy is also called cervical spondylitic syndrome. It is a common and frequently encountered disease in middle-aged and elderly persons. It is reported that approximately 25% of middle-aged and elderly people throughout the world suffer from this problem. Cervical spondylopathy is caused by atrophy of the intervertebral discs or shock absorbers within the neck, narrowing of the cervical intervertebral spaces, or inflammation due to cervical hyperplasia (*i.e.*, bone spurs) that compress the nerve roots in the neck, the vertebral arteries, sympathetic nerve, or spinal cord in the cervical region.

Slight cases of cervical spondylopathy manifest as pain in the head, neck, one or both sides of the shoulders and arms, and numbness in the upper extremities. Severe cases may also manifest aching and weakness in the extremities. In cases with vertebral artery and sympathetic nerve involvement, there may be the symptoms of dizziness and heart palpitations. In the most severe cases where the spinal cord in the cervical region is severely compressed, this may cause fecal and urinary incontinence and paralysis of the extremities.

The treatment of this disease in most cases is non-operative treatment, with massage, including self-massage, as being one of the most effective treatments. Chinese self-massage manipulations can relieve the spasm of muscles and blood vessels in the neck, improve the circulation of blood in the neck, disperse soft tissue swelling, remove adhesions of nerve roots, adjust the relative positions between the intervertebral openings and the nerve roots and blood vessels, and relieve or remove the symptoms caused by stimulation and compression of hyperplasia. From a Chinese medical point of view, Chinese self-massage treats this condition mainly by stimulating and freeing the movement of the qi and blood in the affected area.

**Massage methods:**

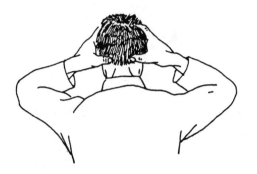

1. Pressing & kneading *Feng Chi* (GB 20): With the tips of both thumbs, press and knead the points just slightly above the posterior hairline in the depression between the mastoid process and the long muscles in the back of the neck 30-50 times. Rotate the head while kneading.

2. Pressing & kneading *Feng Fu* (GV 16): With the tip of the middle finger, press and knead the point 1 body inch above the midpoint of the posterior hairline approximately 100 times.

3. Pushing the *Jia Ji* points (paravertebral points): With the pads of the index and middle fingers of both hands, push the muscles on both sides of the neck from *Feng Chi* downward to the upper back for 1-2 minutes.

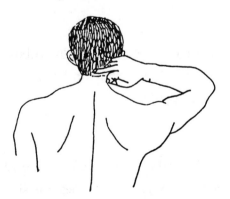

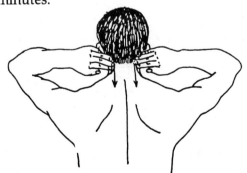

4. Pushing the heavenly pillar bones: With the index and middle fingers of one hand, push the line on the nape of the neck from the midpoint of the hairline to the bulging bone (C7) at the base of the neck 30-50 times.

5. Pinching & grasping the nape: With the thumb, index, and middle fingers of one hand, pinch and grasp the nape of the neck from *Feng Chi* to the base of the neck 30-50 times.

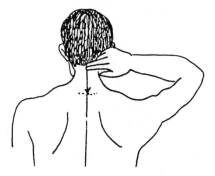

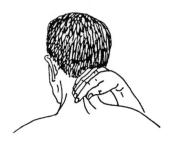

6. Pressing & kneading tender points: With the tip of the thumb or the tips of the index and middle fingers, press and knead any tender point on the neck until the pain is relieved.

7. Pounding the neck: With the side of one fist, lightly pound the back and sides of the neck, shoulders, and upper back 30-50 times. ➜

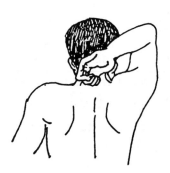

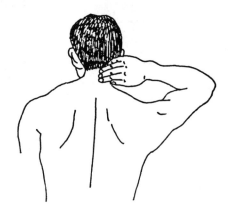

8. Rubbing the neck: With one palm, rub the back and sides of the neck up and down to produce a feeling of heat.

9. Rotation & traction of the neck: Rotate your head in every direction 10-20 times, the size of the circles going from small to large. Then, with

the help of a friend or family member, apply traction to the head upward with one hand holding the chin and the other hand holding the base of the skull. Do this 3-5 times.

10. Grasping & rubbing the arm: With the thumb, index, and middle fingers of the other hand, grasp the outer and inner sides of the affected arm from the shoulder to the wrist several times. Then, with the palm, rub both sides of the arm to produce a feeling of heat.

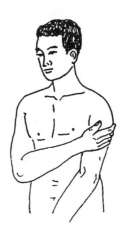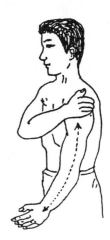

To treat this condition with Chinese self-massage one must persevere. This massage can be done in the morning or the evening. Self-massage should also be combined with movement of the neck, such as lateral flexion, forward flexion, backward flexion, and rotation. One should sleep with a low pillow at night and avoid catching cold, keeping the neck warm.

## 3. Periarthritis of the shoulder

Periarthritis of the shoulder is also called frozen shoulder. In China, it is often referred to as 50 year shoulder since it often occurs in people around 50 years of age. Its main symptoms are pain in the shoulder and impairment of shoulder movement. The rate of occurrence of this disease in females is slightly higher than in males. Most patients with this condition are persons who do physical labor. This disease is an inflammation in the capsule of the shoulder joint and in the soft tissues around the shoulder joint. It is mainly caused by chronic shoulder strain or acute traumatic injury.

Chinese self-massage is quite effective for treating periarthritis of the shoulder. Shoulder movement in most cases can be restored if exercises of the shoulder are carried out in combination with the massage. As with all the conditions in this chapter, Chinese self-massage treats this condition by promoting and freeing the flow of qi and blood in the affected area.

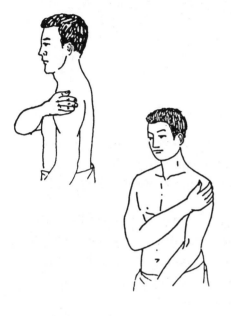

**Massage methods:**

1. Kneading the shoulder: With the heel of the palm of the other hand, knead every side of the affected shoulder beginning with weak pressure and gradually applying stronger pressure for 3-5 minutes.

2. Pinching & grasping the muscles of the shoulder: With the thumb, index, and middle fingers of the other hand, pinch and grasp the muscles of the affected shoulder for 3-5 minutes, grasping more on the deltoid muscle on the lateral side of the shoulder.

3. Pinching & grasping the upper arm: With the thumb, index, and middle fingers of the other hand, pinch and grasp the muscles of the anterior and posterior sides of the affected upper arm from the shoulder to the elbow 30-50 times. ➡

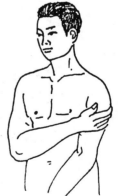

4. Pressing & kneading tender points: With the tip of the thumb or middle finger, press and knead any tender points around the shoulder beginning with weak pressure and gradually pressing more strongly. At the same time, mobilize the shoulder for 2-3 minutes.

**136**

5. Rotating the shoulder joint: Rotate the affected shoulder joint in both directions approximately 10 times. Begin with small circles and increase to large circles.

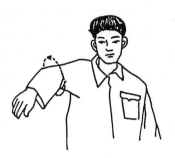

6. Rubbing the shoulder & upper arm: With the other palm, rub every side of the affected shoulder and upper arm to produce a feeling of heat.

**Functional exercises for the shoulder:**

These exercises can be carried out in combination with massage for adhesions of shoulder joint and impaired shoulder movement in the late stage of this condition. Choose from among the following exercises depending on in which direction movement is impaired.

1. Bending the waist & rotating the shoulder: Bend the waist, stretch the arm, and rotate the shoulder joint. The movement should begin small and gradually increase to larger. It should also start off slow and end fast.

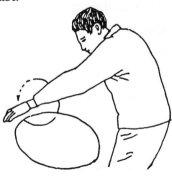

2. Climbing the wall: Stand facing a wall. With the two hands or one hand climbing the wall, raise the arms as high as possible and make a mark on the wall. Then resume one's starting posture. Repeat several times trying to increase the height touched every day.

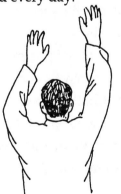

3. Leading the hand behind the body: Bring both hands behind the body. With the healthy hand holding the affected wrist, lead the affected arm backward as far as possible. Do this procedure repeatedly.

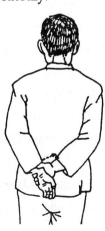

4. Outward rotation exercise: Stand with one's back to a wall. Make fists and flex the elbows. Rotate both arms outward, trying to make the back of the fists touch the wall. Do this procedure repeatedly.

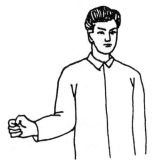

5. Both shoulders adduction & abduction: Cross the hands at the back of the neck and draw in and stretch out the shoulders repeatedly.

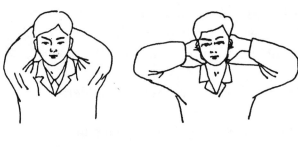

6. Swing the arm movement: Stand upright. Flex the shoulder forward, stretch it backward, and adduct and abduct the shoulder. The size of the movement should go from small to large. Do this procedure repeatedly.

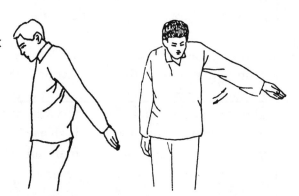

## 4. Tennis elbow

Tennis elbow is also called epicondylitis. Its main symptom is pain in the lateral aspect of the elbow joint which is worse with movements such as rotation, stretching backward, lifting, pulling, holding horizontally, and pushing. This pain radiates downward along the extensor muscle of the wrist on the lateral side of the forearm. It is difficult for the patient to rotate their forearm and to hold things. There may be slight swelling locally and obvious tenderness to palpation on the outside of the elbow.

This disease can be caused by acute sprain of the elbow, but, in most cases, there is no obvious history of sprain. This condition is seen most frequently in adults who often rotate the forearm and stretch the wrist strenuously over and over again, such as tennis players, carpenters, and electricians. This is why it is so called "tennis elbow."

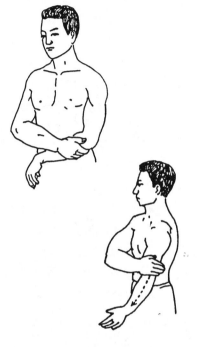

**Massage methods:**

1. Pressing & kneading the lateral side of the elbow and forearm: With the thumb, press and knead the lateral side of the elbow, forearm, and wrist of the affected arm. Repeat this procedure 5-10 times.

2. Pressing & kneading *Qu Chi* (LI 11) and *Shou San Li* (LI 10): With the thumb, press and knead *Qu Chi* (located in the depression at the lateral end of the transverse crease of the elbow when the elbow is flexed) and *Shou San Li* (located 2 body inches directly below the point *Qu Chi*) on the affected arm 30-50 times each.

3. Pressing & kneading tender points: With the thumb, press and knead any tender points on the lateral side of the affected elbow for 2-3 minutes.

4. Elbow motion: Flex and stretch the elbow and rotate the forearm 10-20 times each.

5. Rubbing the lateral side of the elbow and forearm: With the other palm, rub the lateral side of the elbow and forearm on the affected arm to produce a feeling of heat. ➡

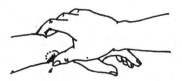

Because this condition is most often the result of repetitive microtrauma, it is absolutely important to rest the affected arm and give the tissues a chance to heal. Although Chinese self-massage can help speed the recovery time, if one immediately reuses the arm again in the same way that caused the problem in the first place, one will never achieve lasting results. This is the only thing difficult about curing tennis elbow.

## 5. Carpal tunnel syndrome

Carpal tunnel syndrome refers to nerve symptoms, such as numbness of fingers, which are caused when the median nerve is compressed in the carpal tunnel of the wrist. Like tennis elbow above, it is most often due to repetitive microtrauma. It is often linked to overuse or wrong ergonomic use of keyboards or "mice" by data entry workers. The carpal tunnel is composed of the wrist bones and transverse carpal ligament which wraps around the carpal bones giving leverage to the muscles of the forearm which control the fingers of the hand. The median nerve and finger flexor tendons pass through this tunnel, and if the tendons swell due to injury or disease, then the median nerve may be compressed within this narrowed space. This then causes the symptoms associated with this syndrome.

At the beginning of this condition, there is numbness in the three and a half fingers on the radial side of the hand. These three and a half fingers are the thumb, index, middle, and half of the ring finger. There may also be numbness in the palm or even in the forearm. If this progresses, there will be loss of sensation in the three and a half fingers and atrophy and weakness of the muscles at the base of the thumb. Thus there may be inability or impaired ability to pick things up. Carpal tunnel syndrome is also statistically more prevalent in women than men.

**Massage methods:**

1. Pressing & kneading the forearm: With the palm of the other hand, press and knead the affected forearm on the palmar side from the wrist to the elbow 5-10 times.

2. Pressing & kneading the points on the forearm: With the thumb of the other hand, press and knead the points *Qu Ze* (Per 3, located in the middle of the transverse elbow crease on the medial side of the tendon), *Nei Guan* (Per 6, located 2 body inches above the midpoint of the transverse wrist crease on the palmar surface of the forearm) and *Yu Ji* (Lu 10,

located at the midpoint between the base of the thumb and the base of the palm on the lateral, palmar side of the hand) on the affected side of the forearm and palm 100-200 times for each point.

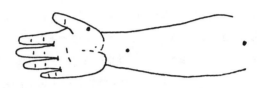

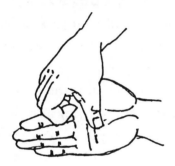

3. Pressing & kneading the area of the carpal tunnel: With the tip of the thumb, press and knead the affected wrist and surface of the palm, beginning with weak force and ending with strong, for 2-3 minutes.

4. Rotation & traction of the wrist: With the other hand, hold the fingers of the affected hand. Then extend the wrist backwards and flex it forward as far as possible approximately 10 times in each direction. Next, rotate the wrist approximately 10 times in each direction and finally pull the wrist straight forward, tractioning it 3-5 times.

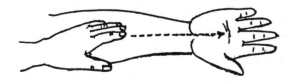

5. Rubbing the palm & forearm: With the other palm, rub the affected forearm from the surface of the palm to the elbow to and fro10-20 times.

**141**

## 6. Acute lumbar sprain

Due to humankind's assumption of an upright posture, more mechanical pressure is applied to the lower back region than most other parts of the body. Therefore, lumbar sprain is a very common complaint in daily life. The main causes of lumbar sprain are carrying heavy objects, trying to lift too heavy objects with the back instead of the legs, sudden twisting of the waist, and injury due to fall or strike directly on or to the low back. For best results, Chinese self-massage should be used as soon after the acute injury as possible. The longer one waits, the more likely that acute lumbar sprain may become chronic low back pain which then is enduring and difficult to treat. Chinese self-massage is a very effective method for treating lumbar sprain. Generally, two to three treatments with Chinese self-massage can cure acute lumbar sprain.

Usually, patients with this complaint experience at least some symptoms immediately after the sprain, such as severe lumbar pain, limitation of and difficulty moving as when sitting, lying, turning over and sitting up from bed, and worsening of the pain when coughing, sneezing, or taking a deep breath. If the case is mild, there may be no obvious lumbar pain immediately after the sprain, but they may experience progressive pain or limited lumbar movement several hours or 1-2 days later.

**Massage methods:**

First one should assume a comfortable position, either sitting or lying on one's side, to help the lumbar muscles completely relax.

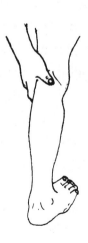

1. Grasping *Wei Zhong* (Bl 40): Place each thumb on *Wei Zhong* (located on the exact midpoint of the transverse crease in back of each knee) and the other fingers on the front of each knee, grasping with five fingers of each hand on *Wei Zhong* of each leg 30-50 times to produce a feeling of mild soreness and distention.

2. Pressing & kneading the lumbar region: With the
heel of one palm, press and knead the lumbar
muscles on the affected side, moving from top
to bottom as one presses and kneads. Do this for
2-5 minutes to help the lumbar muscles to relax.

3. Pressing & kneading tender points: With the tip
of one thumb, press and knead any tender points and
the area around such tender points in the lumbar region.
The force should go from weak to strong but bearable. Continue
pressing and kneading for 2-3 minutes. It is a good sign if this
tenderness is relieved after pressing and kneading these tender points.

4. Rubbing the lumbar region: With
the side of one palm, rub the lumbar
muscles on the affected side up and
down to produce a sensation of heat.
Then, with the center of the palm, rub
the lumbosacral region transversely to
and fro to produce a sensation of heat.
Some massage ointment, such as Tiger
Balm or Temple of Heaven, should be
applied to the area prior to rubbing to
improve the curative effect.

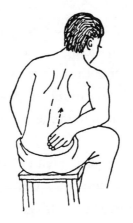
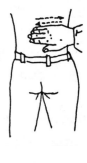

For best results, place a hot compress on the low back region after this self-massage. One can
use several slices of fresh ginger simmered in a pan of water for 5-7 minutes to help move the
qi and quicken the blood. If the back sprain is severe, one should stay in bed resting for 3-4
days, moving the waist as little as possible. In China, it is felt that one should lie on a wooden
bed, *i.e.*, a bed without a mattress. In the West, this means lying on the floor, something that

most low back pain patients instinctively do. Most patients also find that lying on their side in the fetal position gives them the most relief. Acupuncture and Chinese herbal medicine can also help speed recovery from acute lumbar sprain.

## 7. Chronic lumbar muscle strain

Chronic lumbar muscle strain mainly refers to chronic injury of the soft tissues of the low back, such as the muscles, ligaments, and connecting tissue in the lumbosacral region. Chronic low back strain is the main cause of chronic lumbago. Chronic lumbar muscle strain is mainly due to long-term muscle fatigue and repetitive microtrauma, such as from working in an asymmetric or ergonomically inappropriate posture. Chronic lumbar muscle strain may also be caused by acute lumbar sprain which has not been treated soon enough or completely or which has reoccurred many times. Thus acute lumbar sprain may evolve into chronic lumbar muscle strain. In most cases of chronic lumbar muscle strain, there is mild soreness or a vague, lingering pain at ordinary times. This pain then becomes more severe when the person either becomes fatigued or the weather becomes overcast and rainy. This pain may be located on one or both sides or in the middle of the lumbosacral area. The tender area is comparatively large and there are no fixed tender spots. In addition, there is usually no disturbance or limitation in the movement of the waist and low back area.

Treating chronic lumbar muscle strain with Chinese self-massage is less effective than treating acute lumbar sprain. Sometimes, Chinese self-massage does get marked results after several treatments, but unfortunately, this condition may also easily relapse when the person gets fatigued or during cold, damp weather. Thus, in order to be effective, one must persevere in regularly performing Chinese self-massage for the treatment of chronic lumbar muscle strain. Otherwise good effects cannot be obtained.

**Massage methods:**

One should use more force in doing the following Chinese self-massage maneuvers for chronic lumbar strain than that used in treating acute lumbar sprain above.

1. Pressing & kneading the lumbar region: With the heel of each palm, press and knead the lumbosacral muscles on both sides of the low back, moving from top to bottom at the same time as pressing & kneading. Do this for 3-5 minutes to produce a feeling of soreness and distention. The force of pressing and kneading should be deep and strong. (See picture, page 141, #2)

2. Plucking the lumbar muscles: With the tips of both thumbs, press and knead the lumbosacral muscles on both sides of the spine and then pluck the muscles like plucking the string of a guitar, moving from top to bottom at the same time as plucking. Do this for 3-5 minutes.

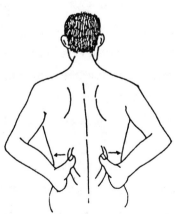

3. Grasping the lumbar muscles: With the five fingers of each hand, grasp the lumbar muscles on both sides of the spine from top to bottom 5-10 times.

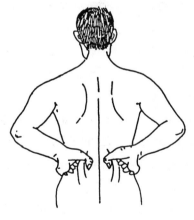

4. Pressing & kneading *Shen Shu* (Bl 23) and *Da Chang Shu* (Bl 25): With the tips of both thumbs, press and knead the paired points *Shen Shu* (located 1.5 body inches lateral to the lower edge of the 2nd lumbar vertebra) and *Da Chang Shu* (located 1.5 body inches lateral to the lower edge of the 4th lumbar vertebra) 100-200 times each point.

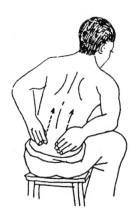

5. Rubbing the lumbosacral region: With both palms, rub the lumbosacral muscles on both sides of the spine up and down to produce a feeling of heat. Then, with one palm, transversely rub the lumbosacral region to and fro to also produce a feeling of heat. One should apply some massage ointment to the area before rubbing.

Doug Frank has written a book titled, *Low Back Pain: Care & Prevention with Traditional Chinese Medicine*, published by Blue Poppy Press. This book has chapters on exercise and low back pain, diet and low back pain, posture and low back, and many other hints and helpful tips on self-treating chronic and acute low back pain. It is a must read for anyone with low back pain who is at all interested in Chinese medicine. When Chinese self-massage is used in conjunction with acupuncture and/or Chinese herbal medicine for the treatment of chronic low back muscle strain, the effects are much better than using any of these alone.

## 8. Knee joint injury

The joints of the knees are among the largest and most complex joints in the body. Because they bear such a heavy burden and are subjected to such a wide variety of forces coming from all different angles, injury of the knee joint is very common. There are several kinds of knee joint injury depending on which tissues within or around the knee have been injured. The most common ones are injury of the collateral ligament, inflammation of the joint capsule due to trauma, and injury of the meniscus of the knee joint. The main symptoms of acute knee joint injury are pain and swelling in the knee joint and restriction of the movement of the knee. In the early stage of injury, Chinese self-massage manipulations should be applied with weak and gentle force to disperse swelling and relieve pain. As the pain and swelling are alleviated, the self-massage can become gradually stronger and small range movement of the knee joint can be gradually added.

## Massage methods:

1. Pressing & kneading the points around the knee joint: With the tip of the thumb, press and knead the points *Xue Hai* (Sp 10, located 2 body inches above the inner, upper border of the kneecap), *Liang Qiu* (St 34, located 2 body inches above the outer, upper border of the kneecap), *Yin Ling Quan* (Sp 9, located in the depression on the lower border of the medial condyle of the tibia), *Yang Ling Quan* (GB 34, located in the depression in front of and below the small head of the fibula), *Xi Yan* (M-LE-16, located in the depressions just below the kneecap on both sides of the patellar ligament), and *Wei Zhong* (Bl 40, located at the exact midpoint of the transverse crease in the back of the knee) 100-200 times each point on the affected side.

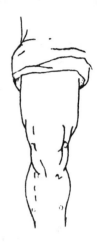

2. Pressing & kneading tender points: With the tip of the thumb, press and knead any tender points found near the knee joint for 3-5 minutes.

3. Pushing & kneading the knee region: With the heel of one palm, knead the area of the knee, moving while kneading from the thigh to lower leg along the anterior, medial, and lateral sides of the knee 3-5 times on each side.

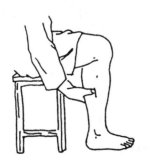

4. Grasping the lower limb: With the five fingers of one hand, grasp the anterior, posterior, medial, and lateral sides of the affected lower limb from the thigh to the foot 3-5 times on each side.

5. Kneading & circular rubbing the injured area: With one palm, gently knead or circularly rub the injured area until a feeling of heat is felt.

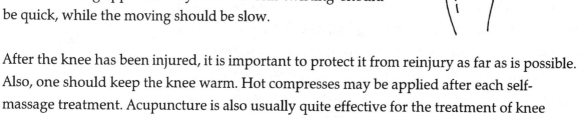

6. Twisting & kneading the knee joint: Place one palms on each side of the affected knee joint, twisting and kneading the knee joint with both palms like twisting a rope. While twisting, move along both sides of the knee from the thigh to the lower leg approximately 10 times. This twisting should be quick, while the moving should be slow.

After the knee has been injured, it is important to protect it from reinjury as far as is possible. Also, one should keep the knee warm. Hot compresses may be applied after each self-massage treatment. Acupuncture is also usually quite effective for the treatment of knee injuries and chronic knee pain.

## 9. Sprained ankle

The ankle joint is the easiest joint in the body to sprain. Most sprained ankles occur when walking on an uneven road, down stairs or on a downhill path, running, or jumping. Eversion or turning outward of the lateral ankle is more common than eversion of the medial ankle. Chinese self-massage is effective for treating sprain or partial rupture of the deltoid ligament. However, Chinese self-massage is contraindicated if there is complete rupture of the ligament, fracture of the ankle bones, or dislocation of the ankle joint. Therefore, if the ankle is severely injured with severe swelling and pain, one should see a professional health care practitioner.

**Massage methods:**

1. Pressing & kneading the points on the lower leg: For sprain of the lateral ankle, press and knead with the thumb on the points *Zu San Li* (St 36, located 3 body inches below the lower,

outside edge of the kneecap), *Jie Xi* (St 41, located at the midpoint of the transverse ankle crease on the back of the foot), *Kun Lun* (Bl 60, located in the depression between the outside ankle and the tendon of the heel), and *Qiu Xu* (GB 40, located in front and below the outside ankle bone), approximately 100 times each point.

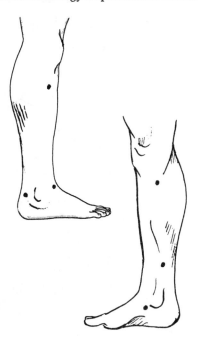

For sprain of the medial ankle, press and knead with the thumb on the points *Yin Ling Quan* (Sp 9, located in the depression on the inferior border of the medial epicondyle of the tibia), *San Yin Jiao* (Sp 6, located 3 body inches above the tip of the inner ankle), and *Shang Qiu* (Sp 5, located in front and below of the inner ankle bone) approximately 100 times each point.

2. Pushing & kneading the lateral or medial side of the lower leg: With the heel of the palm, knead the outer or inner side of the lower leg, moving at the time of kneading from the knee to the ankle 3-5 times on each side of the leg.

3. Grasping the lower leg: With the five fingers of one hand, grasp the lateral or medial side of the lower leg from the knee to the ankle 3-5 times on each side of the leg. (See picture, page 143, #4)

4. Circular rubbing the injured area: With the center of the palm, circularly rub the injured area where it is painful for 3-5 minutes.

5. Rubbing the injured area: With the center of the palm, rub the injured area up and down to produce a feeling of heat. The force of rubbing toward the center of the body should be strong, while the force toward the toes of the foot should be weak so as to subdue swelling.

In other words this rubbing should push body fluids back upward towards the trunk of the body and away from the foot.

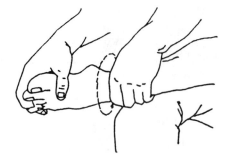

6. Rotating the ankle joint: Hold the tip of the foot in one hand and cup the heel of the foot with the other. Then rotate the ankle clockwise and counter-clockwise 10-20 times in each direction.

7. Tractioning the ankle joint: Hold the foot with both hands in the same way as rotating the ankle joint described above, pulling and extending the ankle joint after rotating it, fully extending the ankle joint 3-5 times.

Do not self-massage the immediately affected area during the first 24 hours after spraining the ankle. Only massage the points on the lower leg at some distance from the swelling and only slightly rotate and traction the ankle. One can apply ice during the first 24 hours and most definitely should keep the leg elevated. After 24 hours, self-massage can be applied directly to the swollen, hot area. Hot compresses after self-massage can also be applied after the first 24 hours and ice should be discontinued since, after the first 24 hours, cold will only restrict the flow of qi and blood in the affected area. Patients should also rest the ankle and not try to walk on it for 3-7 days. When one begins walking on it again after that time, one should use an elastic bandage to provide support. However, when not using the ankle, this bandage should be removed to allow the circulation of the qi, blood, and body fluids. Professional practitioners of Chinese medicine can give emergency first aid Chinese herbs as soon after injury as possible to help minimize swelling and inflammation and thus speed recovery. Acupuncturists may help speed recovery by bleeding the tip of the ankle on the affected side. Instead of hot compresses, professional practitioners of Chinese herbal medicine may prepare herbal soaks or bathes for the foot and ankle.

# Index

# OTHER BOOKS ON CHINESE MEDICINE
# AVAILABLE FROM BLUE POPPY PRESS
3450 Penrose Place, Suite 110, Boulder, CO 80301
For ordering 1-800-487-9296  PH. 303\447-8372 FAX 303\245-8362

**LOW BACK PAIN: Care & Prevention with Chinese Medicine** by Douglas Frank, ISBN 0-936185-66-X

**MASTER HUA'S CLASSIC OF THE CENTRAL VISCERA** by Hua Tuo, ISBN 0-936185-43-0

**MASTER TONG'S ACUPUNCTURE:** An Ancient Alternative Style in Modern Clinical Practice by Miriam Lee 0-926185-37-6

**THE MEDICAL I CHING:** *Oracle of the Healer Within* by Miki Shima, OMD, ISBN 0-936185-38-4

**MANAGING MENOPAUSE NATURALLY with Chinese Medicine** by Honora Lee Wolfe ISBN 0-936185-98-8

**PAO ZHI: Introduction to Processing Chinese Medicinals to Enhance Their Therapeutic Effect,** by Philippe Sionneau, ISBN 0-936185-62-1

**PATH OF PREGNANCY, VOL. I, Gestational Disorders** by Bob Flaws, ISBN 0-936185-39-2

**PATH OF PREGNANCY, Vol. II, Postpartum Diseases** by Bob Flaws ISBN 0-936185-42-2

**PEDIATRIC BRONCHITIS: Its Cause, Diagnosis & Treatment According to TCM** trans by Gao Yu-li and Bob Flaws, ISBN 0-936185-26-0

**PRINCE WEN HUI'S COOK: Chinese Dietary Therapy** by Bob Flaws & Honora Lee Wolfe, ISBN 0-912111-05-4, $12 95 (Published by Paradigm Press)

**THE PULSE CLASSIC: A Translation of the** *Mai Jing* by Wang Shu-he, trans by Yang Shou-zhong ISBN 0-936185-75-9

**THE SECRET OF CHINESE PULSE DIAGNOSIS** by Bob Flaws, ISBN 0-936185-67-8

**SEVENTY ESSENTIAL TCM FORMULAS FOR BEGINNERS** by Bob Flaws, ISBN 0-936185-59-7

**SHAOLIN SECRET FORMULAS for Treatment of External Injuries,** by De Chan, ISBN 0-936185-08-2

**STATEMENTS OF FACT IN TRADITIONAL CHINESE MEDICINE** by Bob Flaws, ISBN 0-936185-52-X

**STICKING TO THE POINT 1: A Rational Methodology for the Step by Step Formulation & Administration of an Acupuncture Treatment** by Bob Flaws ISBN 0-936185-17-1

**STICKING TO THE POINT 2: A Study of Acupuncture & Moxibustion Formulas and Strategies** by Bob Flaws ISBN 0-936185-97-X

**A STUDY OF DAOIST ACUPUNCTURE** by Liu Zheng-cai ISBN 1-891845-08-X

**TEACH YOURSELF TO READ MODERN MEDICAL CHINESE** by Bob Flaws, ISBN 0-936185-99-6

**THE SYSTEMATIC CLASSIC OF ACUPUNCTURE  & MOXIBUSTION** (*Jia Yi Jing*) by Huang-fu Mi, trans by Yang Shou-zhong & Charles Chace, ISBN 0-936185-29-5

**THE TAO OF HEALTHY EATING ACCORDING TO CHINESE MEDICINE** by Bob Flaws, ISBN 0-936185-92-9

**THE TREATMENT OF DISEASE IN TCM, Vol I: Diseases of the Head & Face Including Mental/Emotional Disorders** by Philippe Sionneau & Lü Gang, ISBN 0-936185-69-4

**THE TREATMENT OF DISEASE IN TCM, Vol. II: Diseases of the Eyes, Ears, Nose, & Throat** by Sionneau & Lü, ISBN 0-936185-69-4

**THE TREATMENT OF DISEASE, Vol. III: Diseases of the Mouth, Lips, Tongue, Teeth & Gums,** by Sionneau & Lü, ISBN 0-936185-79-1

**THE TREATMENT OF DISEASE, Vol. IV: Diseases of the Neck, Shoulders, Back, & Limbs,** by Philippe Sionneau & Lü Gang, ISBN 0-936185-89-9

**THE TREATMENT OF DISEASE, Vol. V:**
**Diseases of the Chest & Abdomen,** by Philippe Sionneau & Lü Gang, ISBN 1-891845-02-0

**THE TREATMENT OF EXTERNAL DIS-**
**EASES WITH ACUPUNCTURE & MOXI-**
**BUSTION** by Yan Cui-lan and Zhu Yun-long, ISBN 0-
936185-80-5

**630 QUESTIONS & ANSWERS ABOUT**
**CHINESE HERBAL MEDICINE: A**
**WORKBOOK & STUDY GUIDE** by Bob Flaws
ISBN 1-891845-04-7

**230 ESSENTIAL CHINESE MEDICINALS**
by Bob Flaws, ISBN 1-891845-03-9